Public Health Medicine

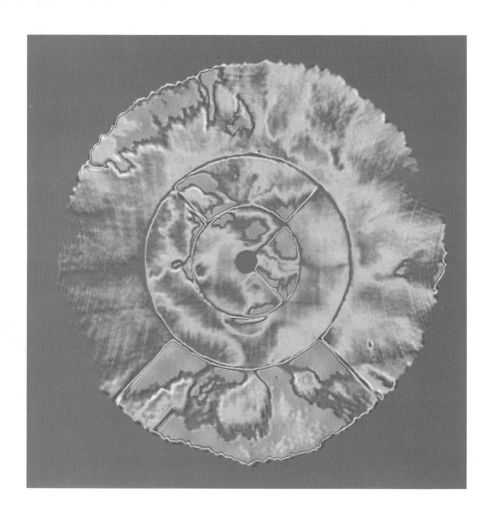

LECTURE NOTES ON

Epidemiology and Public Health Medicine

RICHARD FARMER

MB PhD FFPHM MRCGP
Professor of Public Health
Department of Public Health and Primary Care
Charing Cross and Westminster Medical School
University of London

DAVID MILLER

MD FRCP FFPHM
Emeritus Professor of Public Health Medicine
University of London

ROSS LAWRENSON

MRCGP FAFPHM
Senior Lecturer in Public Health Medicine
Department of Public Health and Primary Care
Charing Cross and Westminster Medical School
University of London

Fourth edition

b

Blackwell
Science

© 1977, 1983, 1991, 1996 by
Blackwell Science Ltd
Editorial Offices:
Osney Mead, Oxford OX2 0EL
25 John Street, London WCIN 2BL
23 Ainslie Place, Edinburgh EH3 6AJ
238 Main Street, Cambridge
  Massachusetts 02142, USA
54 University Street, Carlton
  Victoria 3053, Australia

Other Editorial Offices:'
Arnette Blackwell SA
  224, Boulevard Saint Germain
  75007 Paris, France

Blackwell Wissenschafts-Verlag GmbH
  Kurfürstendamm 57
  10707 Berlin, Germany

  Zehetnergasse 6, A-1140 Wien
  Austria

First published in 1977 under the title
Lecture Notes
on Epidemiology and
Community Medicine
Second edition 1983
Third edition 1991
Fourth edition 1996

Set by Excel Typesetters Co., Hong Kong
Printed and bound in Great Britain
at the Alden Press
Oxford and Northampton

The Blackwell Science logo is a
trade mark of Blackwell Science Ltd,
registered at the United Kingdom
Trade Marks Registry

DISTRIBUTORS

Marston Book Services Ltd
PO Box 269
Abingdon
Oxon OX14 4YN
(*Orders:* Tel: 01235 465500
          Fax: 01235 465555)
USA
Blackwell Science, Inc.
238 Main Street
Cambridge, MA 02142
(*Orders:* Tel: 800 215-1000
          617 876-7000
          Fax: 617 492-5263)

Canada
Copp Clark, Ltd
2775 Matheson Blvd East
Mississauga, Ontario
Canada, L4W 4P7
(*Orders:* Tel: 800 263-4374
          905 238-6074)

Australia
Blackwell Science Pty Ltd
54 University Street
Carlton, Victoria 3053
(*Orders:* Tel: 03 9347 0300
          Fax: 03 9349 3016)

A catalogue record for this title
is available from the British Library

ISBN 0-86542-611-2

Library of Congress
Cataloging-in-Publication Data

Farmer, R. D. T.
    Lecture notes on epidemiology
and public health medicine /
Richard Farmer, David Miller,
Ross Lawrenson.—4th ed.
        p.   cm.
    Includes bibliographical references
and index.
    ISBN 0-86542-611-2
    1. Public health.   2. Epidemiology.
    I Miller, D. L. (David Louis)
    II Lawrenson, Ross.   III Farmer, R. D. T.
    Lecture notes on community medicine.
    IV Title.
    [DNLM: 1. Epidemiologic Methods.
    2. Preventive Medicine.
    3. Health Services.
    WA 950 F234L 1996]
    RA425.F34   1996
    614.4—dc20   95-26229
                                          CIP

Contents

Preface

In order to safeguard and improve the health of society, whatever its stage of development, it is essential to understand why diseases arise. To do this it is necessary to study the distribution and natural history of disease in populations and to identify the agents responsible, so that societies can devise and plan preventive programmes and services for the sick.

The discipline of public health medicine is concerned with these aspects of medical practice. It does not normally involve the diagnosis or management of disease in individual patients. Essentially the subject is concerned with raising the level of health of groups of people and with meeting their collective ambitions for a better quality of life.

In the past, public health medicine and the related basic medical sciences, in particular medical statistics and sociology applied to medicine, did not occupy a major place in undergraduate medical education. This relative neglect of these subjects has changed markedly in the 20 years since *Lecture Notes on Epidemiology and Community Medicine* (as it was then called) first appeared. The GMC's recently published document on *Tomorrow's Doctors: Recommendations on Undergraduate Medical Education* gives fresh impetus to this positive trend. It refers to 'an evident re-awakening of the wider interest of our forebears in the health of populations, the epidemic and environmental hazards that affect them and the means whereby diseases may be controlled or prevented'. It goes on to recommend that 'the theme of public health medicine should figure prominently in the [undergraduate] curriculum, encompassing health promotion and illness prevention, assessment and targeting of population needs, and awareness of environmental and social factors in disease'. This explicit and forceful advocacy for the discipline from a body as influential as the GMC will undoubtedly give added momentum to current developments in medical education. Similar changes emphasizing the importance of disease prevention and the need to ensure that health care is relevant, effective and efficient are evident within the National Health Service in the UK, as in many other countries. This is exemplified in the UK Government's priorities set out in its strategy document, 'The Health of the Nation' and the role accorded to public health medicine in implementing this strategy.

This edition of *Epidemiology and Public Health Medicine* aims to respond to the renewed interest in what our discipline has to offer medical practice and health care services and the resurgent vitality of the discipline. The text has been expanded to take account of new developments, there is much fresh illustrative material and, in addition to some re-organization, there is a new chapter on 'Health Targets' which focuses on the priority conditions identified in 'The Health of the Nation'. Factual information elsewhere in the text has been brought up to date, though the rapidly changing health service structure and sources of health data have made it difficult to keep pace and, in some respects, made it impossible.

We trust that this revised text conveys some of the excitement and rewards that public health offers its practitioners in all health disciplines and that it will continue to serve the needs of both students and teachers, whose comments and suggestions will always be welcome.

Acknowledgements

We are greatly indebted to Dr Norman Begg and Dr Marian McEvoy of the CDSC for their assistance in identifying illustrative material and for kindly providing the data on which a number of graphs and charts are based.

We are also grateful to the many colleagues whose constructive comments have assisted us in this revision.

Richard Farmer
David Miller
Ross Lawrenson

List of Abbreviations Used

AHA   Area Health Authority
AIDS   Acquired immune deficiency syndrome
BCG   Baccille Calmette–Guérin (vaccine)
BMA   British Medical Association
CCDC   Consultant in Communicable Disease Control
CDSC   Communicable Disease Surveillance Centre
CEHO   Chief Environmental Health Officer
DHA   District Health Authority
DoH   Department of Health
DTP   Diphtheria/tetanus/pertussis (vaccine)
FHSA   Family Health Service Authority
GMC   General Medical Council
HEA   Health Education Authority
HIV   Human immunodeficiency virus
HSE   Health and Safety Executive
ICD   International Classification of Diseases
IHD   Ischaemic heart disease
IPV   Injected polio vaccine
MMR   Measles/mumps/rubella (vaccine)
MRC   Medical Research Council
NHS   National Health Service
NHSME   National Health Service Management Executive
OPCS   Office of Population Censuses and Surveys
OPV   Oral polio vaccine
PHLS   Public Health Laboratory Service
PMR   Perinatal mortality rates
RAWP   Resource Allocation Working Party
RCT   Randomized controlled trial
RHA   Regional Health Authority
SMR   Standardized mortality ratio
STD   Sexually transmitted disease
WHO   World Health Organization

PART I

Epidemiology

CHAPTER 1

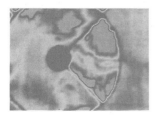

General Principles

The word epidemiology is derived from Greek and means literally 'studies upon people'. Modern methods of epidemiological enquiry were first developed in the course of investigating outbreaks of infectious diseases in the nineteenth century. However, in contemporary medical practice the scope and applications of epidemiology have been greatly extended. Similar methods are now used in the investigation of the causes and natural history of all types of disease. They are also used in the development and assessment of preventive programmes and treatments, and in the planning and evaluation of health services. In contrast to clinical medicine, epidemiology involves the study of groups of people (populations) rather than the direct study of individuals. This does not diminish its relevance to clinical medicine. On the contrary, it enhances the practice of medicine by increasing the understanding of how diseases arise and how they might be managed both in the individual and in societies as a whole.

Most doctors find themselves involved with epidemiology from time to time, in one way or another, either as participants in investigations or through the use they make of the results of studies. It is important that all doctors, and others involved in health care, should have an understanding of the subject so that they can take advantage of opportunities to use epidemiological methods in the study of health and disease and be able to evaluate other people's contributions before accepting their conclusions.

THE INVESTIGATION OF CAUSES AND NATURAL HISTORY OF DISEASE

One of the most important roles of epidemiology is to provide a broader understanding of the causes and natural history of diseases than can be gained from the study of individual cases. Clearly, the experience of an individual doctor is limited because the number of patients with a particular condition with whom he or she comes into contact is relatively small. The less frequent a disease, the more fragmentary is an individual doctor's experience and understanding of it. If the experience of many doctors is recorded in a standard form and properly analysed then new and more reliable knowledge can often be acquired which will assist in diagnosis and point to optimum management policies. Such systematic collection and analysis of data about medical conditions in populations is the essence of epidemiology.

The value of pooling doctors' experience in elucidating the causes of disease is well illustrated by the story of the epidemic of fetal limb malformations (phocomelia) that was caused by pregnant women taking the drug thalidomide during the first trimester. Phocomelia, a major deformity in the development of the limbs, was a recognized congenital abnormality long before the invention of thalidomide. A drawing by Goya called 'Mother with deformed child' bears witness to the fact that it occurred in eighteenth century Spain (Fig. 1.1). However, under normal circumstances it is a very rare abnormality. Any doctor may encounter such rare conditions at some time during their professional life, but, because they know it has already been described, they are unlikely to regard a single case as a noteworthy observation. If, over a short period of time, each of a dozen or so doctors or midwives throughout the country delivered a child with such an abnormality, each would be personally interested but the significance of these individual cases would pass unnoticed unless the doctors or midwives communicated with each other or there was a central reporting system. This is what happened early in the course of the thalidomide episode. One of the lessons learned from the episode was highlighted in the Chief Medical Officer's report of 1966. He said that it '...focused attention on the lack of information concerning the different types of congenital malformations. ... Had a national scheme for notification been available at this time, it is probable that the increase in limb deformities would have been noticed earlier and perhaps some of the tragedies could have been avoided'.

The thalidomide incident underlines the need to collect, collate and analyse data about the occurrence of disease in populations as a matter

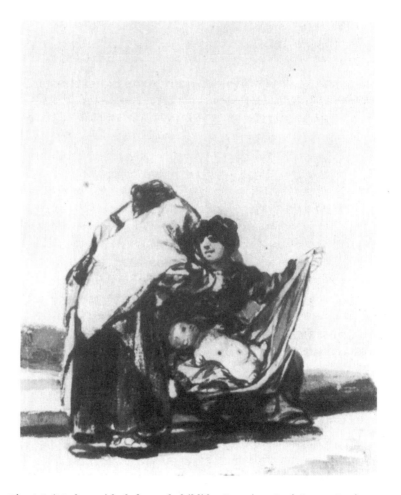

Fig. 1.1 'Mother with deformed child' by Fransisco José Goya y Lucientes. (By courtesy of the Cliché des Musées Nationaux, Paris.)

of routine. This will increase the probability that causes will be identified early and, whenever possible, eliminated. However, even with the most efficient and complete system of recording medical observations, it is unlikely that all problems of cause would be solved. It is interesting to speculate about what would have happened had thalidomide been universally lethal to the fetus before the 12th week of pregnancy. A large number of the spontaneous abortions would have passed unnoticed, some even to the pregnant woman, and the possibility that thalidomide had any deleterious effect on the human fetus would not have come to light. The discovery of such causal relationships requires other approaches, but still depends on the study of populations and cannot be established by examination of individual cases. The same is true for most proposed causes (agents) and other factors which may determine or predispose to the occurrence of disease.

DISEASE IN PERSPECTIVE

Another application of epidemiological techniques is to give perspective to the range of diseases facing doctors and the diversity of their natural history. The individual clinician only sees a selected and comparatively small proportion of sick people, and so may gain an erroneous impression of the relative frequency of different conditions in the community as a whole. He or she may also fail to appreciate the range of different ways in which diseases present and progress. This is important since, consciously or not, the clinician tends to rely on his or her personal experience to assess the likelihood of particular diagnoses and the prognosis in patients when deciding management policy, rather than on unbiased evidence obtained from population studies.

HEALTH CARE NEEDS

Apart from its significance in day-to-day clinical practice, an unbalanced picture of disease incidence or prevalence may also distort the view of the health care needs of the community. In the National Health Service and in most health care systems throughout the world, attempts are now being made to organize services according to priorities set by objective criteria rather than allowing them to be dictated solely by subjective judgements and traditional provision. An important report published in the early 1980s called *Inequalities in Health*, (Townsend & Davidson, 1992) drew attention to some of the major differences that persist in the patterns of illness and disability in England and in the use of health services between different socio-economic groups. For example, men in social class V were reported to suffer from long-standing illnesses almost twice as often as those in social class I but they consulted their general practitioner only about 25% more often. This observation suggests a serious failure to match needs with appropriate services. It calls for detailed investigation of the relevant population groups to elucidate the reasons for it and the implications for future health care provision.

EVALUATION OF MEDICAL INTERVENTIONS

Finally, epidemiology is of value in testing the usefulness (and safety) of medical interventions. Although many existing remedies have never been subjected to trial, everyone nowadays recognizes the necessity to conduct clinical trials of a new drug or vaccine before it is introduced into medical practice. This is the only way to demonstrate that a particular drug or vaccine is likely to improve the patient's prospects of recovery or to prevent disease from occurring or progressing. Once a product has been launched on the market it is necessary to continue to monitor its effects (both beneficial and adverse) in order to ensure that patients are being prescribed effective and safe medication. In recent years, the role of epidemiology, which is exclusively concerned with the application of epidemiological methods to the assessment of medicines, has become firmly established.

It is now accepted that the same principles ought to be applied to other treatments, such as surgery or physical therapy, and even to the alternative ways in which health services can be provided. Such trials are becoming increasingly numerous, but they usually need to be on a large scale to produce reliable results. This is expensive and time consuming but necessary in the long-term interests of health care.

CLINICAL MEDICINE AND EPIDEMIOLOGY

It will be clear from the above that there are important contrasts between the approaches to disease by clinicians and by epidemiologists. Recognition of these differences helps understanding of the subject. The clinician asks the question 'What disease has my patient got?' The epidemiologist asks 'Why has this person rather than another developed the disease? How could it be prevented? Why does the disease occur in winter rather than summer? Why in this country but not in another?' In order to answer such questions it is necessary to compare groups of people, looking for the factors that distinguish people with disease from those without. Underlying the investigation of disease in this way is the belief that the misfortune of an individual in contracting a disease is not due to chance or fate but to a specific, definable and preventable combination of circumstances.

For a clinician, the utility of a diagnosis is a pointer to management decisions. Therefore the diagnostic precision required is related to the specificity of treatments that are available. For an epidemiologist, diagnosis has different significance. It is a way of classifying individuals in order to make comparisons between groups. Lack of precision leads to poorly defined categories. This makes it difficult to identify the subtle yet important differences between groups which are critical to the understanding of the causes and prevention of disease.

The clinician is interested in the natural history of disease for prognostic purposes in an individual patient. He or she is usually content to express prognosis in terms such as 'good', 'bad', 'about 6 months', etc. It is unhelpful to the clinician and the patient to attempt to introduce mathematical precision into prognostic statements, such as 'He has a 10.9% chance of surviving symptom-free for 5 years', though it may sometimes be appropriate to give a range of expected survival times, for example between 3 and 7 years. By contrast, in population studies precision is helpful because it may allow the investigator to identify variables that have significant effects on outcome. For example, it may be informative to investigate why in one group of patients 10.9% survive symptom-free for 5 years while in another group with approximately similar conditions, 26.5% survive symptom-free for 5 years. What accounts for this difference which could assist in planning treatment or preventive strategies?

While there are these clear differences between clinical and epidemiological approaches to medical problems and while their immediate purposes are different, it is also clear that the results of epidemiological investigations can contribute greatly to the scientific basis of clinical practice.

CHAPTER 2

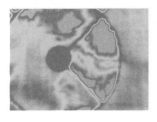

'Cause' and 'Risk' and Types of Epidemiological Study

INTRODUCTION

The principal uses of epidemiology in medicine have been described in Chapter 1. These can be summarized as:

• the investigation of the causes and natural history of disease, with the aim of disease prevention and health promotion;

• the measurement of health care needs and the evaluation of clinical management, with the aim of improving the effectiveness and efficiency of health care provision.

Both involve two important and fundamental concepts—*cause* and *risk*. The concept of *cause* must be distinguished from the notion of *association*. Not all factors that are statistically associated with the occurrence of disease are causes. They also include so-called 'determinants', confounding variables and factors associated by pure chance.

CONCEPT OF CAUSE

• A *cause* is an external agent (microbe, chemical substance, physical trauma) which results in disease in susceptible individuals.

• A *determinant* is an attribute or circumstance that affects the liability of an individual to be exposed to or, when exposed, to develop disease, e.g. hereditary predisposition, environmental conditions.

• A *confounding variable* is a factor which is significantly associated with both the occurrence of a disease in a population and with one of its causes or determinants, but is not itself a cause. For example, heavy cigarette smoking and a high alcohol consumption tend to occur together. Smoking is causally associated with carcinoma of the bronchus and because heavy drinking is associated with cigarette smoking, alcohol consumption will tend to correlate with carcinoma of the bronchus, even though it is not a cause.

The concept of *risk* includes both the 'risk' that a person exposed to a potentially harmful agent will develop a particular disease and the 'risk' that a particular intervention will beneficially or adversely influence the outcome. The indices commonly used to measure risk are set out below.

Risk factors are different but are involved in both concepts. They are factors that are associated with a particular disease or outcome. They can be associated either by chance or because they influence the course of events. All causal agents and determinants are 'risk factors' but not all 'risk factors' are causal agents or determinants.

The purpose of epidemiological studies is to identify causes and determinants and to define and measure risks by the application of the scientific methods set out in the next four chapters.

CAUSES AND DETERMINANTS

Few diseases have a single 'cause'. Most are the result of exposure of susceptible individuals to one or more causal agents. Even in the case of some of the most straightforward illnesses, for example infections, exposure to the causal agent does not inevitably result in disease. Many other factors may influence the development of disease in addition to the direct cause. Thus, the investigation of cause is usually a complex exercise that involves both the identification of the characteristics of susceptible individuals (and sometimes characteristics of individuals who appear to be unusually resistant) and the types of exposure to external agents that are necessary for the disease to occur.

Ideally, causal hypotheses should be explored by carefully controlled experiments in which the effects of each of the postulated causes can be examined independently of other factors. In animal studies, for example, it is usually possible to exclude the effects of inheritance by breeding a family of animals for study. The possible effects of the general environment and diet that are not of interest for a particular investigation can be eliminated by rearing the whole family under standard conditions. Then the effects of a suspected causal agent can be assessed by exposing a sample of the animals to it whilst protecting others from it. In such experiments the only major difference between the two groups is their exposure to the agent under study. Such a study design allows the observed effects, if any, to be attributed unequivocally to the agent under investigation. It is impractical and unethical to undertake studies of such experimental purity amongst human subjects. The identification of the causes of diseases and factors that alter the course of a disease in humans necessitates adopting methods whereby hypotheses can be tested without prejudice to the individuals being studied.

The methods that are used in epidemiological studies represent practical compromises of the above 'ideal' design. It is essential, therefore, that the results of any investigation are interpreted in full knowledge of the limitations imposed by the compromises. In particular, it is important to take account of the effects of confounding variables and, when these cannot be controlled in the study design, to allow for them in the analysis.

Distinguishing causes and determinants from chance association

The observation that a disease is statistically associated with a suspected agent is clearly not proof that the suspected agent causes the disease. For example, there is a higher prevalence of alcoholism amongst publicans and bar staff than in most other occupational groups. This does not necessarily mean that being a publican causes alcoholism. There are several other possible explanations of this phenomenon, including the fact that people who tend to excessive alcohol consumption may seek jobs in bars.

The types of evidence that can be used to distinguish a causal from a fortuitous association are discussed below. Many of the criteria appear to be simple and straightforward but it can be seen that each of them can present practical difficulties.

DISTINGUISHING CAUSE FROM ASSOCIATION

- Strength of association
- Time sequence
- Distribution of the disease
- Gradient
- Consistency
- Specificity
- Biological plausibility
- Experimental models
- Preventive trials

STRENGTH OF ASSOCIATION

The stronger the association the more likely it is to be causal. This is usually measured in terms of relative risk, i.e. the incidence of disease in people exposed to the suspected agent compared with the incidence in those not so exposed (see below).

TIME SEQUENCE

If an agent causes a disease then exposure must always precede its onset. A practical problem is that it is often difficult to date exposure to a suspected causal agent and the date of onset of the disease. For example, AIDS is usually not manifest until many years after infection with HIV. Most people with AIDS could have become infected with HIV on many occasions. By the time the disease is apparent it is impossible to prove that a particular exposure or type of activity led to the infection.

DISTRIBUTION OF THE DISEASE

The spatial or geographical distribution of the disease should be similar to that of the suspected causal agent. This may be difficult to demonstrate, particularly if there is a significant time interval between exposure and manifestation of disease and there have been movements in the population during that interval. For example, legionnaires' disease commonly occurs in people who become infected as a result of casual or transient exposure to the source and who may be widely scattered before they develop symptoms of the disease.

GRADIENT

The incidence of disease should correlate with the amount and duration of exposure to the suspected cause (population dose–response). For example, mesothelioma was noted to be more common than expected in people working with asbestos and in those living near to factories which emitted asbestos dust into the atmosphere. The incidence was greatest in workers exposed for the longest periods and those living in closest proximity to the factories. In many instances, however, it may be difficult to quantify exposure.

CONSISTENCY

The same association between a disease and a suspected causal agent should be found in studies of different populations. Failure to find consistency may be explained by differences in study design. Caution is needed before rejecting a causal hypothesis in such circumstances. For example, studies designed to test the hypothesis that carcinoma of the breast is causally associated with exposure to oral contraceptives have produced conflicting results. Some appear to demonstrate that women exposed to oral contraceptives over long periods of time have an increased risk of breast cancer under the age of 35 years; others do not support this hypothesis. Careful review of the studies reveals differences in the criteria for the selection of cases and in the analytic techniques used, which may explain the apparently conflicting results. A causal hypothesis can be regarded as supported only when there is a general consistency of findings from studies conducted in the same way.

SPECIFICITY

The disease should occur only in people exposed to the suspected agent. This criteria is of particular use with infectious diseases. For example, the disease typhoid fever occurs only in patients infected with *Salmonella typhi*. For many non-infectious diseases, such as cancer and heart disease, there are often multiple causes of the same condition.

BIOLOGICAL PLAUSIBILITY

The association between the disease and exposure to the suspected causal agent should be consistent with the known biological activity of the suspected agent. Sometimes an association is observed before the biological process is identified. The fact that there is no known biological explanation for an association should not lead to rejection of a biological hypothesis. For example, in the mid-nineteenth century, John Snow suggested that cholera was caused by an invisible agent in water. The epidemiological data were entirely consistent with the hypothesis but the cholera vibrio and its mode of spread had yet to be discovered.

EXPERIMENTAL MODELS

The disease can be reproduced in experimental models with animals. The fact that exposure to an agent can produce a disease in animals similar to that seen in humans gives credence to a causal hypothesis, but failure to produce the disease amongst animals cannot be used as evidence to reject the hypothesis. For example, some micro-organisms are pathogenic in humans but not usually in animals, e.g. measles virus; others are pathogenic in animals but not usually in humans, and only a minority are normally pathogenic in both.

PREVENTIVE TRIALS

Control or removal of the suspected agent results in decreased incidence of disease. For example, when it was appreciated that the use of thalidomide for treatment of morning sickness in pregnancy was associated with a high incidence of phocomelia, the drug was withdrawn and the epidemic rapidly ceased.

RISK

There are three common indices of risk: absolute, relative and attributable.

> ### TYPES OF RISK
>
> *Absolute*: incidence of disease in any defined population
> *Relative*: ratio of the incidence rate in the exposed group to the incidence rate in the non-exposed group
> *Attributable*: difference between the incidence rates in the exposed and non-exposed groups

Absolute risk

This is the most basic measurement; it is the incidence of a disease in any defined population. The absolute risk in an exposed population taken in isolation is not a very useful index because it assumes that there is no risk of the disease in people who are not exposed to the agent. It is more useful, therefore, to quantify the relationship between the risk of the disease amongst those exposed to the agent under investigation and those not so exposed.

Relative risk

This is the ratio of the incidence rate in the exposed group to the incidence rate in the non-exposed group. It is sometimes expressed as a percentage. It is a measure of the proportionate increase (or, if the agent is protective, the decrease) in disease rates of the exposed group. Thus, it makes allowance for the frequency of the disease amongst people who are not exposed to the supposed harmful agent.

Attributable risk

This is the difference between the incidence rates in the exposed and the non-exposed groups, i.e. it represents the risk attributable to the factor being investigated.

The use of these measures of risk can be illustrated with data collected during the course of a cohort study which compared mortality amongst cigarette smokers with non-smokers during a 7-year period (Table 2.1).

MORTALITY OF SMOKERS VS. NON-SMOKERS			
	Number in study	Died within 7 years	Death rate over 7 years (per 1000)
Cigarette smokers	25 769	133	5.16
Non-smokers	5 439	3	0.55

Table 2.1 A comparison of mortality amongst cigarette smokers and non-smokers.

Absolute risk in cigarette smokers = 5.16 per 1000
Relative risk in cigarette smokers = 5.16/0.55 = 9.38
Attributable risk of cigarette smoking = 5.16 − 0.55 = 4.61 per 1000

This indicates that smokers were 9.38 times more likely to die during the 7-year period than non-smokers and that the additional risk of death carried by smokers compared with non-smokers was 4.61 per 1000 people per 7 years. The confidence with which these findings can be applied to the general population is determined in part by the similarity of the two groups in respect of attributes other than their smoking habits, in part upon whether the smokers are representative of the whole population of smokers and in part upon the sizes of the samples investigated. If the sampling was truly representative, the proportion of deaths in smokers that would be eliminated by cessation of smoking is the ratio of attributable to absolute risk (4.61/5.16 = 89%). This is known as the *attributable fraction*.

TYPES OF EPIDEMIOLOGICAL STUDY

There are four broad types of epidemiological study:
- descriptive;
- cohort;
- case–control;
- intervention.

They serve different purposes. None of them is entirely clear cut and it is not profitable to try to classify each and every study within these classical types. Frequently the detailed investigation of a disease involves undertaking several studies of different types. They are defined and explained here to enable the reader to understand the concepts involved and to provide a framework which can be used to identify the most

appropriate study design to answer particular problems. They are discussed in greater detail, with examples, in ensuing chapters.

Descriptive studies

These are used to demonstrate the patterns in which diseases and
associated factors are distributed in populations. They aim to identify
changes in mortality and morbidity in time or to compare the incidence
or prevalence of disease in different regions or between groups of
individuals with different characteristics (e.g. occupational groups). Cor-
relations are then sought with one or more other factors which may be
thought to influence the occurrence of the diseases. Studies of this type
may give rise to hypotheses of cause but cannot be used in isolation to
explore the meaning of associations and can rarely prove cause. This
requires the use of the other types of study.

Cohort and case–control studies

These are planned investigations designed to test specific hypotheses.
They aim to define the causes or determinants of diseases more precisely
than is possible using descriptive studies alone. From the results, it is
often possible to suggest ways whereby the disease may be prevented or
controlled. Both cohort and case-control studies rely on data collected in
a systematic manner according to well-defined procedures.

• In a *cohort* investigation individuals are selected for study on the basis
that they are or may be exposed to the agent under investigation and are
readily identified and 'followed-up' for a period of time. The follow-up
may extend into years and aims to identify the characteristics of those
who develop the disease and those who do not.

• The subjects investigated in a *case–control* study are generally recruited
because they already have the disease being investigated. Their past
histories of exposure to suspected causal agents are compared with
those of 'control' subjects—individuals who are not affected with the
disease but are drawn from the same general population. The analysis
involves discriminating between the past exposures and other relevant
characteristics of the cases and those of the controls.

The differences between these two study designs are schematically represented in Fig. 2.1. The cohort study design is closest to the 'ideal'
experimental design. Such studies tend to take longer and to be more
expensive than case–control studies. However, they usually yield more
robust findings. Case–control studies, though usually cheaper and

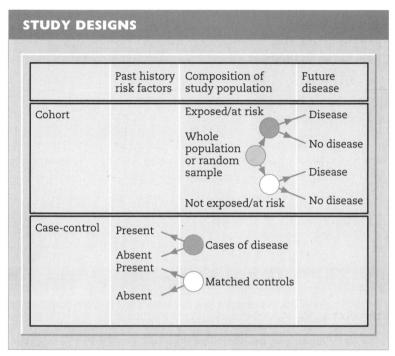

STUDY DESIGNS

	Past history risk factors	Composition of study population	Future disease
Cohort		Exposed/at risk	Disease
		Whole population or random sample	No disease
			Disease
		Not exposed/at risk	No disease
Case-control	Present		
		Cases of disease	
	Absent		
	Present		
		Matched controls	
	Absent		

Fig. 2.1 Comparison of cohort and case–control study designs.

quicker to complete than cohort studies rarely give clear-cut proof of cause.

Intervention studies

These are essentially experiments designed to measure the efficacy and safety of particular types of health care intervention including studies of treatment, prevention and control measures and the way in which health care is provided. They can also be used to assess the comparative effectiveness and efficiency of different interventions. The most familiar study design of this type is the clinical trial. Ethical considerations are important when considering the design and execution of any kind of intervention study.

CHAPTER 3

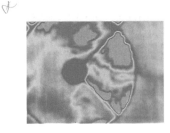

Descriptive Studies

INTRODUCTION

An important starting point for many epidemiological investigations is the description of the patterns of distribution of disease in populations (descriptive studies). The principal advantages of descriptive studies are that they are cheap, quick to complete and they give a useful initial overview of a problem that may point to the next step in its investigation.

Usually, descriptive studies make use of routinely collected health data, for example death certification data, hospital in-patient statistics or infectious disease notifications. The main sources of routine health data are set out in Chapter 8. The social and other variables in relation to which disease data may be examined are also available from a wide variety of routine sources. The actual source used for a particular investigation depends on the data that are required. With the exception of census material, routine sources of social data are not discussed in detail in this book.

Often the data required to describe disease distribution in a population and related variables are not readily available or are unsatisfactory for epidemiological purposes. In these circumstances it is necessary to conduct special surveys in order to collect the raw material for a descriptive study. These surveys are usually cross-sectional in type (see Chapter 4).

USE OF DESCRIPTIVE STUDIES

Aetiological

The results of descriptive studies usually only give general guidance as to possible causes or determinants of disease, for example where broad geographical differences in prevalence are shown. Sometimes they may be quite precise, for example where a particular disease is very much more frequent within an occupational group. Analysis of the data may indicate that certain attributes or exposures are more commonly found amongst people who have the disease than in those who do not. The converse may also be demonstrated, namely that certain attributes are more commonly found amongst people who do not have the disease than in those who do. This may be an equally valuable finding. It is not possible to prove that an agent causes a disease from a descriptive study, but investigations of this type will often generate or support hypotheses of aetiology and justify further investigations.

Clinical

Clinical impressions of the frequency of different conditions and their natural history are often misleading. The clinical impression is influenced by the special interests of individual doctors, by events that make a particular impression and by the chance clustering of cases. To obtain a balanced view of the relative importance of different conditions, their natural history and the factors that affect outcome requires data from a total population or an unbiased (random) sample. Precise knowledge of the relative frequency of different diseases at different times and in various situations, and the normal distribution of physiological measurements in particular groups of people is helpful to the clinician in his or her judgement of probabilities when deciding on the most likely diagnosis in individual patients.

Service planning

Health service planning in the past has been largely based on historical levels of provision and responses to demands for medical care. In order to plan services to meet needs rather than demand, and to allocate resources appropriately, accurate descriptive data are required on the relative importance and magnitude of different health problems in various segments of the community. They are also essential in order to evaluate the effectiveness of services and to monitor changes in disease incidence which may indicate a need for control action or the re-allocation of resources and adjustments to service provision.

ANALYSIS OF DESCRIPTIVE DATA

Data derived from routine mortality and morbidity statistics (and from cross-sectional surveys) are usually analysed within three main categories of variable:

- time (when?);
- place (where?);
- personal characteristics (who?).

Time

Three broad patterns of variation of disease incidence with time are recognizable. These are shown below.

VARIATION OF DISEASE WITH TIME

- Long-term (secular) trends
- Periodic changes (including seasonality)
- Epidemics

LONG-TERM (SECULAR) TRENDS

These are changes in the incidence of disease over a number of years that do not conform to an identifiable cyclical pattern. For example, the secular trend in mortality from tuberculosis in England and Wales has shown a steady fall over many years (Fig. 3.1). The observation of this trend on its own does not give any indication of its cause. However, it is sufficiently striking to justify specific studies aimed at trying to identify the reasons for the change. The inclusion in the figure of the times at which various discoveries were made or specific measures were introduced gives some enlightenment. The overall trend seems to have been hardly affected by the identification of the causal organism, or the introduction of chemotherapy and BCG vaccination. This suggests that these played little part in the decline in mortality. However, the presentation of these data on an arithmetic scale (as in Fig. 3.1) disguises an important feature of the trend, i.e. a change in the rate at which the decline occurred. When the data are plotted on a logarithmic scale (Fig. 3.2) it becomes clear that the introduction of specific measures for the control and treatment of tuberculosis was associated with an acceleration in the established de-cline in mortality. It is now thought that the decline in mortality from tuberculosis was due to a complex series of changes. Until the 1950s, these were mainly an increase in the resistance of the population to

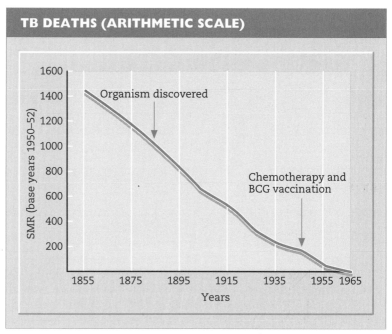

Fig. 3.1 Tuberculosis mortality in England and Wales, 1855–1965 (arithmetic scale).

infection and environmental changes that reduced the chances of acquiring infection. After the early 1950s, the rate of decline in mortality was accelerated by the newly available methods of management.

It is frequently necessary to examine secular trends both as changes in rates (arithmetic scale) and as rates of change (logarithmic scale), if the nature of a trend is to be fully appreciated.

The secular trend in mortality from carcinoma of the bronchus shows the opposite picture to that for tuberculosis (Fig. 3.3). Until quite recently it had been increasing relentlessly amongst males but the rate of increase has now declined. By contrast the increase in mortality rates amongst women continues. The powerful correlation between mortality and changes in the national consumption of cigarettes gave rise to the hypothesis that cigarette smoking could be the causal agent, although it did not prove causality. The hypothesis has since been explored through large numbers of epidemiological studies.

PERIODIC CHANGES

These are more or less regular or cyclic changes in incidence, the most common examples of which are seen in infectious diseases. For example,

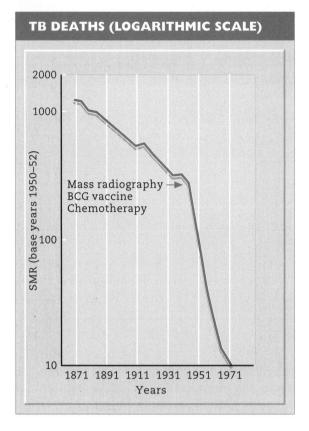

TB DEATHS (LOGARITHMIC SCALE)

SMR (base years 1950–52)

2000
1000

100

10

Mass radiography →
BCG vaccine
Chemotherapy

1871 1891 1911 1931 1951 1971

Years

Fig. 3.2 Tuberculosis mortality in England and Wales, 1871–1971 (logarithmic scale). (Reproduced with permission from HMSO: *Prevention and Health: Everybody's Business*, 1976.)

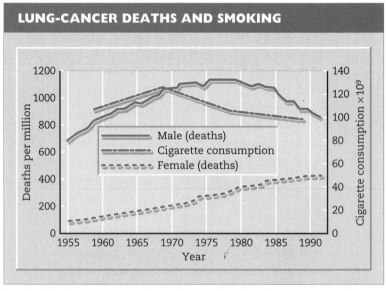

LUNG-CANCER DEATHS AND SMOKING

Deaths per million

1200
1000
800
600
400
200
0

Cigarette consumption ×10^9

140
120
100
80
60
40
20
0

—— Male (deaths)
— - — Cigarette consumption
⚬ ⚬ ⚬ Female (deaths)

1955 1960 1965 1970 1975 1980 1985 1990

Year

Fig. 3.3 Carcinoma of lung, bronchus and trachea. Deaths per million population in England and Wales, 1955–92, and cigarette consumption per year. (Reproduced with permission of the Office of Population Censuses and Surverys (Crown copyright).)

until a vaccine was introduced, measles showed a regular biennial cycle in incidence in England and Wales (Fig. 3.4). The cycles were probably the result of changes in the levels of child population (herd) immunity (see p. 152). Other infectious diseases such as whooping cough, rubella and infectious hepatitis show less regular, but nevertheless distinct, cycles with longer intervals between peaks.

Seasonality

This is a special example of periodic change. The environmental conditions that favour the presence of an agent, and the likelihood of its successful transmission, change with the seasons of the year. Respiratory infections, which spread directly from person to person by the air-borne route, are more common in winter months when people live in much closer contact with each other than in the summer. By contrast, gastrointestinal infections, which spread by the faecal–oral route, often through contamination of food, are more common in summer months when the ambient temperatures favour the multiplication of bacteria in food. The regular seasonality of gastrointestinal infections is shown in Fig. 3.5 in which the number of notifications of food poisoning for each quarter in 1974–89 are plotted. A particularly interesting feature of food

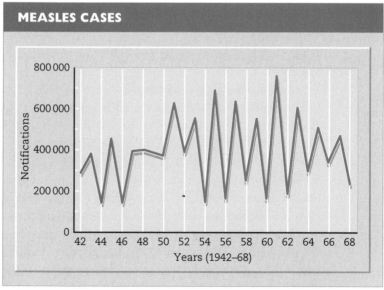

Fig. 3.4 Notifications of measles in England and Wales showing periodic variation (prior to introduction of measles vaccination). (Reproduced with permission of the Office of Population Censuses and Surveys (Crown copyright).)

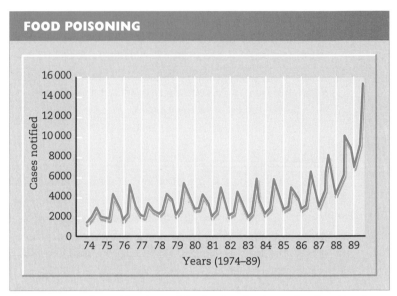

FOOD POISONING

Fig. 3.5 Quarterly notifications of food poisoning in England and Wales, 1974–89.

poisoning incidence is that the marked seasonality is combined with a noticeable secular trend. The number of cases notified from late 1988 and early 1989 was much higher than in previous years. This could be due to contamination in the food chain, a decline in standards of food storage, distribution or preparation, or the result of an increase in notification rates following publicity given to the problem of food poisoning.

Some non-infectious conditions, for example allergic rhinitis, deaths from drowning and road accidents, also display distinct seasonality. For most of these, the explanation for the seasonality is not difficult to infer. There are seasonal variations in the incidence of certain other conditions, however, for which there is as yet no rational explanation. For example, schizophrenic people are more likely than the general population to be born in the early months of the year (February and March) (Table 3.1). Many hypotheses have been offered to explain this observation, including the proposition that the disease is caused by an intra-uterine infection, that the mothers of schizophrenic people are more likely to miscarry at certain times of the year (thereby resulting in a deficit of births in months other than February and March) and that the mothers are more likely to conceive in April and May than are other women. However, none has yet been proved.

It should be noted that the seasonality in disease patterns related to climatic conditions is reversed in the southern hemisphere.

SEASONALITY OF BIRTH AND MENTAL ILLNESS				
	Quarter of birth			
	Jan–Mar	Apr–June	July–Sept	Oct–Dec
Schizophrenic people				
Observed	1383.0	1412.0	1178.0	1166.0
Expected	1292.1	1342.8	1293.1	1211.1
Observed as a percentage of expected	107	105	91	96
Neurotic people				
Observed	3085.0	3172.0	2949.0	2882.0
Expected	3024.1	3150.6	3042.0	2844.2
Observed as a percentage of expected	101	101	97	101

Table 3.1 Seasonality of birth of schizophrenic and neurotic people compared with that of the general population (expected) showing an increased frequency of births of schizophrenic people in the first part of the year but no seasonality amongst neurotic people. (Adapted from Hare E, Price J, Slater E. *Br J Psychiat* 1974; **124**: 81–86.)

EPIDEMICS

These are temporary increases in the incidence of disease in populations. The most obvious epidemics are of infectious diseases such as influenza (Fig. 3.6) but non-infectious epidemics do occur. For example, there was an increase in asthma deaths in the 1960s associated with the increased use of pressurized aerosol bronchodilators (Fig. 3.7, p. 27).

The word 'epidemic' is also sometimes used to describe an increase in incidence above the level expected from past experience in the same population (or from experience in another population with similar demographic and social characteristics). However, if the strict definition of epidemic is used, it is inappropriate to use the term to describe recent secular trends in coronary heart disease, lung cancer or even AIDS, since there is no evidence that any of them are temporary increases in incidence.

Place

Variations in the incidence or prevalence of disease by place can be considered under three headings.

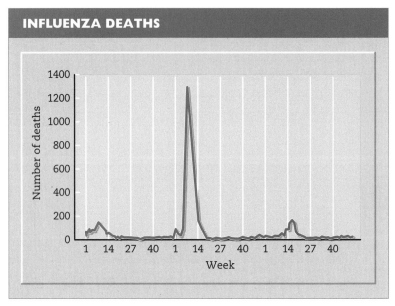

Fig. 3.6 Weekly deaths from influenza in England and Wales, 1975–77.

VARIATION OF DISEASE BY PLACE

- Broad geographical differences
- Local differences
- Variations within single institutions

BROAD GEOGRAPHICAL DIFFERENCES

Variations in the incidence of disease are sometimes related to factors such as climate, social and cultural habits (including diet), the presence of vectors or of other naturally occurring hazards. Although the incidence of disease does not respect administrative boundaries between countries or regions, these boundaries often follow broadly natural ecological boundaries and tend to encompass common social and cultural groups. Much valuable information pointing to possible causes of disease has been obtained by comparisons of routinely collected data between countries and other administrative units. For example, various forms of cancer and other conditions show striking geographical difference in incidence (Table 3.2).

LOCAL DIFFERENCES

The distribution of a disease may be limited by the localization of its cause. Thus, if a main water supply becomes contaminated, the illnesses

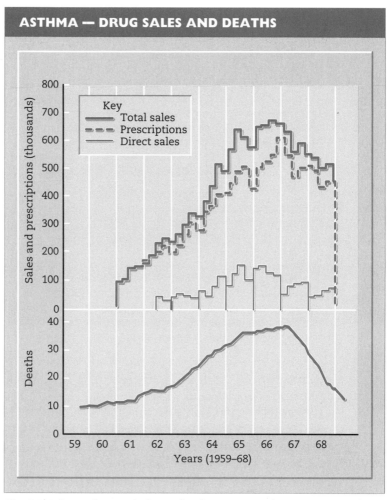

ASTHMA — DRUG SALES AND DEATHS

Fig. 3.7 Sales and prescriptions of asthma preparations compared with deaths from asthma among people aged 5–34 years, in England and Wales, 1959–68. (After Inman WHW, Adelstein AM. *Lancet* 1969; ii: 279.)

that result from the contamination will be clustered in people living within the distribution area of the water. 'Spot-maps' on which cases are marked may show local concentrations which suggest possible sources. In interpreting such maps, it is important to relate the spatial distribution of cases to the density of population. The classical study of the 1854 cholera outbreak in the Golden Square area of London by John Snow used such a technique and led him to identify the particular water pump that was the source of the infection. In this instance, cases were clustered in the streets close to the Board Street pump, while

GEOGRAPHICAL VARIATION IN DISEASE RATES			
		Rates per 100 000	
	Disease	England and Wales	Japan
England and Wales high, Japan low	Cancer of breast (females)	47.9	6.6
	Cancer of prostate	20.2	2.9
	Cancer of colon	20.9	6.3
England and Wales low, Japan high	Cancer of stomach	23.0	43.8
	Cirrhosis of liver (males)	5.0	21.1
	Suicide	8.5	18.0

Table 3.2 Geographical variation in the incidence of disease. Comparison of death rates in England and Wales with those in Japan (1979) for various causes shows considerable discrepancies. Both are highly industrialized countries with well-developed health services, but have very different cultures and racial origins. (Data from World Health Statistics Annual, WHO, Geneva 1981.)

comparatively few cases occurred in the vicinity of other pumps in the area.

A special kind of locality difference is that which exists between urban and rural environments. In general, people who live in urban areas are subjected to different hazards from those experienced by people who live in rural areas. These differences alter their risk of certain diseases, sometimes to the advantage of the country person and sometimes to the benefit of the town dweller. In urban areas, there may be better housing and sanitation but more overcrowding and air pollution; more leisure but less exercise, fresh food and sunlight; more industrial hazards but fewer risks of infection from animal contacts and vectors. In industrial societies, however, where commuting is a common practice, the distinction between town and country dwellers is often blurred. Table 3.3 shows some differences in mortality between urban and rural areas in England and Wales.

VARIATIONS WITHIN SINGLE INSTITUTIONS

In institutions such as schools, military barracks, holiday camps and hospitals, variations in attack rates by class, platoon, chalet or ward may focus attention on possible sources or routes of spread. For example, in

URBAN/RURAL MALE DEATHS

| | | Urban with populations | | | |
| | | Over 100 000 | 50 000– 100 000 | Under 50 000 | |
	Conurbations				Rural
Malignant neoplasms of bronchus, trachea					
and lung	118	109	98	90	79
bladder	112	109	99	96	82
Chronic rheumatic heart disease	114	110	88	94	85
Ischaemic heart disease	99	106	107	101	95
Influenza	84	98	90	116	111
Bronchitis	117	109	98	96	76
Motor vehicle accidents	87	95	98	99	124
Accidental poisoning	126	110	100	89	67
Homicide	151	99	95	71	56

Table 3.3 Differences in mortality amongst males between urban and rural districts in England and Wales 1969–73 (SMRs).

an outbreak of surgical wound infection, identifying the bed positions of patients, ward duties of staff and theatres used may suggest the identity of a carrier or other source of infection. Similarly, in places of work the danger of developing disease may be shown to be inversely related to distance from source of a chemical hazard.

A high incidence of a disease amongst people who share the same environment does not prove that a factor within the environment was the cause of the disease. It may be that the people have chosen, or have been chosen, to share the same environment because they have an increased susceptibility to that disease or because of pre-existing disease or disability.

Personal characteristics

The chances of an individual developing a disease may be affected by personal characteristics. The analysis of data on the incidence of disease in relation to the personal characteristics of victims provides useful indicators of possible causes. The personal characteristics can be classified as shown below.

VARIATION OF DISEASE DUE TO PERSONAL CHARACTERISTICS

Intrinsic factors (affect susceptibility if exposed to causal agents)
- Age
- Gender
- Marital status
- Ethnic group

Personal habits or lifestyle (affect exposure)
- Family
- Occupation and socio-economic group

INTRINSIC FACTORS
Age

Most diseases vary in both frequency and severity with age. In general, children are more susceptible to infectious diseases, young adults are more accident prone and older adults tend to suffer the results of long exposure to occupational and other environmental hazards. In infancy, immaturity and genetic defects affect susceptibility to disease. In later life, physiological changes, degenerative processes and an increased liability to malignant tumours are the dominant determinants of the patterns of illness.

The fact that the incidence of most diseases varies with age can complicate the comparison of morbidity and mortality between populations with dissimilar age structures. For example, the age structure of a population of military personnel is likely to be substantially different from that of a group of practising physicians. Therefore, it is to be expected that the two groups will differ in their incidence of many diseases. In order to make a valid comparison between these populations it is essential to adjust the data to take account of differences in their age structure. This procedure is called standardization (see Chapter 9).

Age differences in the incidence of disease may also be accounted for by a so-called 'cohort effect'. This occurs when individuals born in a particular year, or living at a particular point in time, are exposed to the same noxious agent. They then carry an enhanced risk of the disease caused by that noxious agent for a long period, sometimes for the rest of their lives. For example, the children who were exposed to radiation in Hiroshima and Nagasaki in 1945 when the atomic bombs were detonated have had higher than expected incidence of leukaemia throughout their lives.

Gender

There is evidence that males are intrinsically more vulnerable to disease and death than are females. This is first apparent in the differential rates of stillbirth and early neonatal mortality, and remains throughout life (Table 3.4). Indeed, during later life, with the exception of disorders that are specific to the female, there are few diseases which have a greater incidence in women than in men. In most societies, men are exposed to a greater number and variety of hazards than are females often because of differences in their leisure and work activities. Even when the two sexes are exposed to the same hazards for the same period of time, there is evidence that women are less likely to develop disease and that they survive better than men. Some diseases appear to vary in incidence between the sexes only because they are more readily diagnosed in one sex than the other, for example gonorrhoea in men, or because they are more likely to come to medical attention, for example in mothers of young children.

Marital status

Morbidity and mortality from many diseases vary considerably according to marital status. In most cases both are higher amongst single people. There are two reasons for this. Firstly, marriage is not random. People with pre-existing disabilities or disease are less likely to marry than those without. Thus, individuals so affected will be over-represented in the single (never married) population. Secondly, there are differences between the lifestyles of married and non-married people which affect their

MALE/FEMALE DEATH RATES		
Age	Males	Females
Stillbirths	5.35	4.68
Under 28 days	5.81	4.39
Under 1 year	5.50	3.87
1–4 years	0.44	0.40
5–14 years	0.22	0.17
15–24 years	0.77	0.31
25–34 years	0.87	0.47
35–44 years	1.67	1.12
45–54 years	5.27	3.23
55–64 years	16.60	9.25
65–74 years	42.89	23.44
75–84 years	101.07	62.53
85 years and over	214.71	171.00

Table 3.4 Death rates at different ages for males and females in England and Wales, 1988 (deaths per 1000).

exposure to causal agents, for example sexual behaviour, contact with children, leisure activity and diet. The incidence of some diseases and health problems is higher amongst divorced and widowed people than amongst married people, for example suicide and certain types of mental illness. It is always important to distinguish diseases and exposures that may have determined the marital status of an individual from those that are determined by the marital status.

Ethnic group

This term tends to be used very loosely to describe a number of personal characteristics, including some that are strictly genetically determined, for example skin colour, and some that have nothing to do with genetics, for example country of birth and religion. It is often difficult to disentangle these ethnic characteristics from a number of other factors which affect the incidence of disease, for example dietary habits, religious practices, occupation and socio-economic status. The effect of ethnicity on the incidence of disease is best studied in communities where people of different groups are living side by side and in similar circumstances. For example, studies in the UK have shown a higher prevalance of Type 2 diabetes in Asians compared with the white population. This is probably due to genetic differences. On the other hand, in New Zealand the differences in the cot death rate between Maoris and Europeans is related principally to the lower socio-economic status of most Maoris and lifestyle factors such as maternal smoking.

PERSONAL HABITS OR LIFESTYLE
Family

Some diseases are especially frequent in certain families because of a common genetic inheritance, which is an intrinsic characteristic of the individuals. The risk of disease among members of the same family may also be increased because the members share a common environment and culture. Culture affects a wide range of disease-related factors such as type of housing, dietary habits and the way in which food is prepared, as well as the individual's reaction to illness.

Occupation and socio-economic group

Some people are exposed to special risks in the course of their occupation. These include exposures to dust (particularly coal dust, silica and asbestos), toxic substances and gases used in industrial processes, and the risks of accident. Some occupations influence habits such as the amount of tobacco smoked and of alcohol consumed or the regularity of meals, which in turn affect disease incidence.

When interpreting any observed correlation between occupation and disease it is necessary to take account of the factors which determine a person's choice of occupation. Some may affect the person's susceptibility to disease, for example tall and powerful people may choose physically demanding occupations whilst others may chose 'sheltered' occupations because they already suffer mentally or physically disabling diseases. Some, because of chronic disease, may be unable to keep demanding jobs in the higher socio-economic groups; they tend to move down the social scale (social class migration).

The social class of men and single women is defined in terms of their occupation and their status within an occupational group (i.e. manager, foreman, unskilled). The social class of married women and of children is determined by the occupation of the husband (father). The concept of social class encompasses income group, education and social status, as well as occupation. Most diseases show a positive social class gradient, with a higher incidence in manual workers than in professional groups (Table 3.5).

Interactions of time, place and personal characteristics

Frequently, two or more factors correlate with the incidence of a disease and also with each other. It may be that only one factor is a causal agent or determinant and that the correlation with a second factor is fortuitous. Sometimes, however, two separate causes of disease interact with

DEATH TRENDS BY SOCIAL CLASS						
Cause of death (ICD number)	I	II	IIIN	IIIM	IV	V
Malignant neoplasm of stomach (151)	50	66	79	118	125	147
Malignant neoplasm of trachea, bronchus and lung (162)	53	68	84	118	123	143
IHD (410–414)	88	91	114	107	108	111
Cerebrovascular disease	80	86	98	106	111	136
Bronchitis, emphysema and asthma (490–493)	36	51	82	113	128	188

Table 3.5 SMRs for ages 15–64 years (England and Wales) showing trends by social class for specific causes of death.

each other in such a way that the effect of the two acting together in the same individuals is greater than that of either acting alone. For example, while people who work with asbestos and who do not smoke have a higher incidence of bronchial carcinoma than other non-smokers, those who smoke have a much higher incidence than would be expected in people with similar smoking habits in the general population. Interactions such as this are often very complex and the analysis of observed distributions can do no more than indicate possible determinants which merit more detailed and carefully controlled enquiry. Time, place and personal interactions can be separated if circumstances arise in which one of the variables can be kept constant while the others change. For example, comparison of disease frequency in migrant populations with the frequency in their place of origin is often informative, particularly where migrants move from an area with a high incidence of disease to one with a low incidence, or vice versa. When they migrate, they take with them their original hereditary susceptibilities but they change their risk of exposure to harmful agents. For example, the incidence of cancer of the stomach is higher in Japanese living in Japan than those living in the USA, while for cancer of the large bowel the reverse is true. In time, when migrants are assimilated into the host culture, they may be exposed to new risks in that culture. Thus, studies of migrant groups can also be used to measure the latent period between exposure and onset of disease. For example, the incidence of multiple sclerosis is higher in Europeans who migrated to South Africa before the age of 15 than in those born in South Africa.

It must be stressed that caution is needed in studies of migrants because they are self-selected from the original population and their risks of disease may have been different from those who did not migrate.

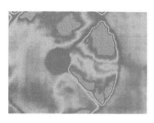

Surveys, Survey Methods and Bias

INTRODUCTION

Many descriptive studies make use of routinely collected data. However, such data are often unsatisfactory for this purpose and specifically designed surveys are needed. The problems are shown below.

PROBLEMS WITH ROUTINELY COLLECTED DATA

PROBLEMS

- Difficulties in ascertainment of cases
- Variations in diagnostic criteria
- Absence of records of the attributes of individuals
- Unsuitable format of records
- Inconsistency in data presentation

Difficulties in ascertainment of cases

The recorded number of patients with a condition may vary for reasons that have nothing to do with the actual frequency of the disease. For example, the tendency to seek medical attention and the availability of services may vary. This source of bias is of greatest importance when studying illnesses that are rarely fatal and therefore do not appear on death certificates, or that are not always medically managed or reported and therefore do not come to the attention of the medical profession.

Example: Osteoarthritis is neither fatal nor is it always treated or reported. Studies of that disease based entirely on the cases treated in hospital or brought to the attention of the general practitioner are misleading.

Variations in diagnostic criteria

These tend to vary between doctors and may change with time. This may be simply a matter of fashion or because the facilities for accurate diagnosis vary. Sometimes, there may be internationally agreed changes in classification practices.

Example: The ICD is revised about every 10 years and some diagnostic categories may not be carried forward from one revision to the next.

In addition the diagnosis may involve a measurement that is not made routinely and/or recorded for the whole of the population.

Example: It is extremely difficult to study the epidemiology of hypertension in the community without doing special surveys because blood pressure is not a measurement that is routinely recorded in the population as a whole. By contrast, birth weight can be studied in some detail because all newly born babies are weighed and their weight is usually recorded.

Absence of records of attributes of individuals

The attributes of the individuals which the study proposes to investigate in relation to the presence of disease may not be recorded systematically.

Example: The occupation of patients is often not recorded or not recorded in sufficient detail in hospital notes to allow investigation of a cancer which it is suspected may result from occupational exposure to a carcinogenic agent.

Unsuitable format of records

The data are recorded but are not usable because the form of the record is unsuitable, or because they are governed by strict rules of confidentiality.

Example: Diagnoses may be recorded but not in a form or in sufficient detail to allow classification by ICD or other standard criteria.

Inconsistency in data presentation

In the analysis of deaths, the numbers and the date of occurrence are indisputable in countries where death registration is standard practice. However, when analysing morbidity by time, there are several possible points of reference. Those commonly used are the date of onset of the disease, the date of onset of symptoms, the date of first diagnosis or the date of hospital admission. In acute diseases, where these points are close together, it does not matter very much which is chosen, but in the case of chronic diseases the intervals may be months or even years. In such circumstances the reference point must be stated and be consistent.

The above difficulties with routinely available data can be partly overcome by well-designed routine information systems. Nevertheless, this cannot meet all requirements and many of the problems can only be overcome by surveys in which the data and means of collection are specified in advance and in which the study population is clearly defined.

CROSS-SECTIONAL (PREVALENCE) SURVEYS

A cross-sectional (prevalence) survey is simply a descriptive study which, instead of relying on routine sources of data, uses data collected in a planned way from a defined population. The aim is to describe individuals in the population at a particular point in time in terms of their personal attributes and their history of exposure to suspected causal agents. These data are then examined in relation to the presence or absence of the disease under investigation or its severity with a view to developing or testing hypotheses as described in Chapter 3.

Example: A cross-sectional survey was carried out among a multiracial workforce at worksites in New Zealand by Scragg and colleagues between 1988 and 1990. The survey studied 5677 staff aged 40–64 years. The subjects were asked about their age, ethnicity, past medical history, occupation and income. Their height, weight and blood pressure were recorded and an oral glucose tolerance test to detect diabetes mellitus

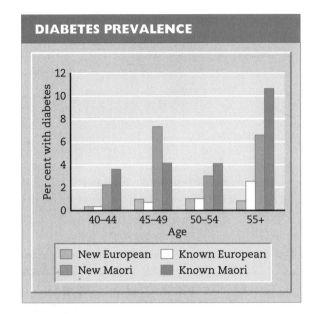

DIABETES PREVALENCE

Fig. 4.1 The prevalence of diabetes both known and previously undiagnosed in Maori and European workers. (From Scrugg R. *et al. NZ Med J* 1991; **104**: 395–7.)

was performed. The study showed that the prevalance of diabetes increased with age, was more common in Maoris and that approximately 50% of workers with diabetes were previously undiagnosed (see Fig. 4.1). The prevalence of diabetes was also significantly correlated with weight and low income.

SURVEY METHODS

A number of practical and theoretical problems can arise in the design and conduct of cross-sectional surveys and other studies which may invalidate the results unless they are handled properly. The investigator needs to be aware of these potential problems and familiar with the methods that are available to solve them or to minimize their effects.

Sampling

It is usually unnecessary to study the whole of a population in order to obtain useful and valid information about that population. The investigation of a sample has many practical advantages. In particular it reduces the number of individuals who have to be interviewed, examined or investigated. It is also often easier to obtain high response rates and high-quality information on smaller numbers. This is always preferable to poor-quality data on larger numbers. If a sample is used, it is essential to ensure that the individuals included in the sample are genuinely representative of the population being investigated–the 'parent' population. There are many methods availabe for selecting a sample. Some commonly used sampling techniques are detailed below.

TYPES OF SAMPLE

- Simple random sample
- Systematic sample
- Stratified sample
- Cluster sample
- Multistage sample

Simple random sample

In this sample each individual in the parent population has an equal chance (probability) of being selected. One way of obtaining a random sample is to give each individual a number and then to use a computer-generated table of random numbers to decide which individuals should be included.

Systematic sampling

This form of sampling is more convenient and is adequate for most purposes. People are selected at regular intervals from a list of the total population. It has the advantage of being easy for field workers to use.

Example: If a one in 10 sample of school children is required then every 10th child on the school role could be included. In some circumstances this method can lead to bias, for example when the school roll (or similar list) is compiled by class (or other grouping), which may affect randomness.

Stratified sample

In this sample the probability of an individual being included varies according to a known and predetermined characteristic. The aim of this method is to ensure that small sub-groups which are of particular interest to the investigator are adequately represented.

Example: If one of the attributes being investigated in a cross-sectional study of school children is the consequences of being an immigrant to the country and immigrants comprise only 5% of the population, then a simple random sample would produce a group in which 5% are immigrants. Unless the sample is very large, the number in the group may be insufficient for a conclusive analysis. To avoid this problem, the sample has to be weighted in favour of the selection of immigrant children. This is done by drawing separate random samples from amongst immigrant and indigenous children, e.g. 50% of immigrants and 10% of the indigenous group. Thus, all immigrant and all indigenous children have equal chances of selection although the chance of an immigrant being selected is greater than the chance of a locally born child being selected. When the data are analysed, the fact that the sample was recruited in this way must be taken into account.

Cluster sample

This involves the use of groups as the sampling unit rather than individuals, e.g. households, school classes or residents within blocks on a grid map. The groups to be studied should be randomly selected from all possible groups of the same type, for example a random sample of all households in England as in the General Household Survey undertaken routinely by OPCS. All members of the selected groups are included in the study. The underlying assumption is that the individuals belonging to any particular group do so for reasons unconnected with the disease being studied and the presence of any factor under investigation. The main advantage of this method of sampling is that the field work is concentrated and, therefore, simpler and cheaper. The principal disadvantage is that diseases and associated factors themselves may have determined the group to which individuals belong which the investigator may not suspect.

Multistage sampling

This combines the above sampling techniques. For example, a series of 'clusters', say schools, might be identified and a random sample of them selected. Then within each school, a random sample of pupils stratified by class would be recruited to the study.

Bias in sampling

There are five important potential sources of bias in selecting any sample.
1 Any deviation from the rules of selection can destroy the randomness of the sample. One of the most common temptations is to recruit volunteers to the study. This is in effect self-selection of participants and such individuals tend to be unrepresentative of the parent population.
2 Bias is introduced if people who are hard to identify in the parent population under study are omitted from the study. Thus, in investigating the health of school children the omission of children who are persistent

absentees may seriously bias results if the reason for their absence is chronic illness.

3 The replacement of previously selected individuals by others can easily introduce bias. If, for example, it proves difficult to trace a person who has been selected or if that person refuses to cooperate, it is not acceptable to replace him or her with an easily traceable or cooperative individual. Replacement of a selected individual is acceptable only if it transpires that they were included in the sample in error, for example a selected subject was subsequently found not to satisfy study criteria.

4 If large numbers of individuals in the sample refuse to cooperate in a study, the results may be meaningless. Therefore, it is essential to make intensive efforts to enlist the cooperation of and trace all the individuals who have been sampled.

5 If the list of people used as a sampling frame is out of date, bias will be introduced owing to omission of recent additions and the inclusion of people who have departed.

ERROR IN RATES

The analysis of epidemiological survey data usually entails the calculation of rates, for example incidence and prevalence rates, in exposed and non-exposed population groups. Rates may be affected by errors and bias in either the numerator or the denominator or both. Such errors can invalidate comparisons between rates, and result in misleading conclusions.

Error and bias in numerator data

The quality of numerator data is crucial for accurate classification of individuals according to their personal attributes, their exposure to suspected causal agents and whether or not they have the disease under investigation. In contrast to descriptive studies based on routine data, special surveys offer the investigator the advantage of being able to specify the observations that he or she wishes to be made, rather than being constrained by the data that are collected for other purposes. Furthermore, the investigator can prescribe the methods to be used in examining or questioning the individuals involved in the study. However, the investigator usually only has a single opportunity to make the observations on each subject. It is therefore essential that the information required is clearly defined at the outset and that efforts are made to ensure that consistent results are obtained by the instruments (questionnaires, laboratory or other measuring equipment) used. Without clarity of definition in the design of the study and consistency in its execution, errors will occur (see below).

ERROR AND BIAS IN NUMERATOR DATA

- Subject variation
- Observer variation
- Limitations of the technical methods used

Subject variation

Differences in observations made on the same subject on different occasions may be due to many factors, including those outlined below.

- Physiological changes in the parameter observed, for example blood pressure, blood glucose.
- Factors affecting the response to a question, for example recollection of past events, motivation to respond and mood at time of interview, reaction to environment and rapport with interviewer.
- Induced changes because the subject is aware that he or she is being studied. (This is sometimes referred to as the Hawthorne effect.)

Observer variation

The principal types of observer variation are as follows.

- Failure of the same observer to record the same result on repeated examination of the same material (inconsistency)–this is called intra-observer variation.
- Failure of different observers to record the same result – this is called interobserver variation. The greater the number of different observers, the greater are the chances of variation between them.

Either of the above types of error can arise for several reasons.

- Bias induced by awareness of the hypothesis under investigation, for example in a study of HIV infection, the observer may probe answers to certain questions more deeply if the subject has declared himself to be a homosexual or an intravenous drug user.
- Errors in executing the test or variations in the phrasing of a question, for example failure to be consistent in the use of a procedure, careless-ness in setting up instruments or reading a scale, failure to follow instructions when administering a questionnaire, omission of some ques-tions or tests, errors in recording of results.
- Lack of experience or skill, and idiosyncrasies of observers, especially when classification depends on a subjective assessment, for example

misinterpretation by the interviewer of an answer to a question, lack of skill in the manipulation of instruments, poor motivation, lack of interest in the project.

• Bias in the execution of the test, for example preconception of what is 'normal' or 'to be expected', digit preference (i.e. tendency to 'round off' readings to whole numbers, fives and 10s) inflection of voice in asking questions.

LIMITATIONS OF THE TECHNICAL METHODS USED

Technical methods may give incorrect or misleading results for the following reasons.

• The test does not measure what it is intended to measure, for example the presence of albuminuria in pregnancy, for which there are many causes, is a poor index on its own of the presence of toxaemia. There-fore, a study of toxaemia in which cases are identified solely by albuminuria will give misleading results.

• The method used is intrinsically unreliable or inaccurate, and thus yields results that are not repeatable or correspond poorly with those obtained by alternative methods, or do not correlate well with the severity of the condition being measured, for example peak flow rate in asthma.

• Faults in the test system, for example defective instruments, erroneous calibration, poor reagents, etc.

Avoidance of numerator error and bias

There are no hard and fast rules that can be applied to ensure that errors do not arise in surveys and that bias is avoided. Each project will require careful thought and consideration of where errors and bias might arise. Some of the more straightforward principles are given below.

• The criteria used in diagnostic classification must be clearly defined and rigidly adhered to (even at the risk of missing a few cases). The features that must be present (or absent) for a diagnosis to be made must be specified.

• Classification of severity or grade of disease should be in quantitative terms where possible and it should cover the full range of possible types of case.

• All subjects should be observed under similar biological conditions on each occasion. Avoid uncomfortable circumstances. Design simple questions and use check questions for consistency of response.

• The number of observers used should be kept to a minimum. They should be trained properly to enhance their skills and test their variation on dummy subjects (or specimens). Take duplicate readings and record the mean value. Arrange for the classification to be re-assessed by different observers, for example independent assessment of histopathology specimens by more than one pathologist.

• Where possible, subjects and observers should be unaware of (blinded to) the specific hypothesis under investigation in order that they are not influenced by personal perceptions of the significance of the variables being recorded.

• The tests selected should be relevant to the purpose. Those that give the most consistent results and are least disturbing to the subject are preferable.

• Equipment should be simple, reliable and easy to use.

• Test methods should be standardized by, for example, the use of standard reagents, sets of graded X-rays or slides, standard wording of questions and instructions on probing and interpretation of answers, and calibration of instruments against a standard reference. Quality control should be maintained to avert 'drift' from standards.

Error and bias in denominators

Errors occur when the population being investigated is not fully defined. Such errors can be minimized by making every effort to encourage cooperation of the potential subjects and avoiding any inconvenience or discomfort to them. All available means should be used to trace and persuade non-attenders to take part or continue to participate in the investigation. The similarity of those who participate and those who are lost from the study should be checked by comparing their general attributes such as age, marital status, sex and occupation to establish how representative they are of the total sample.

There are several ways of handling people lost to follow-up in the analysis phase of an investigation.

• Exclude them from both the numerator and the denominator.

• Include them up to the time that they left. This involves calculating units of 'time at risk' (see p. 48).

• Include all those 'lost' for half the 'time at risk' on the assumption that the rate of loss was even throughout the period and on average each individual was present for half the time.

• Analyse the data on the assumption that all those lost developed the disease, or had the most adverse outcome, and then on the assumption that none of them developed it. This will show the range within which the true result might lie.

Assessment of error in surveys

Some terms that are frequently used in the assessment of error in surveys are given below.

COMMON TERMS IN SURVEY ERROR

- Random error
- Systematic error
- Discrimination
- Reproducibility, assessed by:
    replication of tests
    comparison of test systems
    use of check questions
    random allocation of subject to interviewer
- Validity

RANDOM ERROR

This is due to the chance fluctuation of recorded values around the 'true' value of an observation.

SYSTEMATIC ERROR (BIAS)

This is a consistent difference between the recorded value and the 'true' value in a series of observations. For example, if the height of an individual is always measured when the person is wearing shoes, then the measurement will be consistent but will have a systematic bias.

DISCRIMINATION

This relates to whether a test is able either to separate people with a disease (or a particular attribute) from those without the disease (or attribute) or to place subjects accurately on a range of severity (or a scale measuring an attribute). The degree to which this is achieved correctly is a measure of discrimination. A test with good discriminatory power has a small range of error in relation to the potential range of true results. There are two basic characteristics of a test which measure its discriminatory powers: its *reproducibility* and its *validity*.

REPRODUCIBILITY (RELIABILITY, REPEATABILITY)

This is a measure of the consistency with which a question or a test will produce the same result on the same subject under similar conditions on successive occasions. A highly reproducible test must have low random error, although it may still have systematic error.

When reproducibility is evaluated by retesting subjects, it is usually defined as the ratio of the number of cases positive on both occasions to the number positive on at least one occasion. It can be assessed by the following procedures.

• Replication of tests. The results of a series of measurements by the same observer or by different observers using the same test on the same group of subjects (or set of specimens) under identical conditions are compared.

• Comparison of test systems. The measurements are repeated using a different instrument or test system. Statistical analyses can be used to identify whether the variation is attributable to the test system, intra-observer variation, interobserver variation or subject variation. Similar methods can be applied to the assessment of the reproducibility of questions, but there are problems because when the same question is repeated, the subject (and observer) may be conditioned by replies given on previous occasions.

Other procedures for assessing the reproducibility of questionnaires:
• the use of check questions, i.e. questions which seek the same information though in a different form, for example age and date of birth;
• the random allocation of subjects to different interviewers and comparing results between groups.

VALIDITY (ACCURACY)

This is a measure of the capacity of a test to give the true result. A valid test is one that correctly detects the presence or absence of a condition or places a subject correctly on a scale of measurement. For example, glycosuria as a test of the presence of diabetes has poor validity compared with a glucose tolerance test.

Validity has two components. In the case of a test which divides a population into two groups, validity is assessed by how well it picks up those with diseases (its *sensitivity*) and how well it rejects those without disease (its *specificity*) (see p. 209).

CHAPTER 5

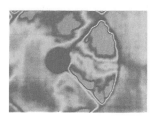

Cohort Studies

INTRODUCTION

Cohort studies involve the investigation of groups of people who have no manifestations of the disease under study at the time they are recruited. The selected study group is observed over a period of time in order to measure the frequency of occurrence of the disease amongst people exposed to the suspected causal agent compared with its frequency amongst individuals who are not exposed. Cohort studies can be used in a similar way to identify the determinants of disease in the study population.

TYPES OF COHORT

- Groups with special personal characteristics
- Groups with special exposures

GROUPS WITH SPECIAL PERSONAL CHARACTERISTICS

Groups of individuals who have special characteristics unrelated either to their risk of exposure or to their risk of disease, and which make them easy to follow-up, provide useful cohorts for the investigation of many diseases. Cohorts that have been used because they are easy to study over long periods of time include, for example, those selected because they belong to a profession of which a register is constantly maintained (e.g. doctors, nurses, etc.); individuals who are members of a particular insurance scheme; or employees in industries with a low turnover of workers.

At the time of recruitment to the study, the investigator identifies the characteristics of the subjects by the use of standard questionnaires or the measurement of any number of biological variables. They are then followed up until a sufficient proportion have reached a predefined end point (usually the development of the disease being investigated or death). During the follow-up period, their exposures to suspected harmful agents are recorded. Such cohorts can be used to estimate prevalence, incidence and risk in relation to a suspected causal agent without recruiting an additional comparison (control) group because the comparison group (those not exposed to the agent being investigated) is a sub-group of the cohort itself. This is called an internal control group.

GROUPS WITH SPECIAL EXPOSURES

The other main type of cohort comprises groups of individuals who have all been exposed to the agent or the experience that is being investigated. This type of cohort requires the concurrent recruitment and study of an external control group. The control group in this instance must be drawn from a population that is similar to the exposed group in all respects other than their exposure to the agent under investigation. The data on the control group must be the same and collected in the same way as those on the exposed group.

These two types of cohort study can be equally valuable in epidemiological studies. The choice depends on the question being studied and the availability of suitable study populations.

TIME AT RISK

In an ideal situation, all members of either type of cohort are recruited to a study at about the same time and followed up for the same period of time. Sometimes, it is not possible to recruit sufficient numbers to yield significant results in a short period, particularly if exposure to the agent or the disease being investigated is relatively rare. Moreover, in most studies, some patients are lost to follow-up. Either situation will result in variations in the length of time during which individual members of cohorts are observed. This gives rise to problems in the analysis of the data.

One way to handle variations in the periods during which individuals have been observed is to use the total time at risk in each group as the denominator. It is calculated by summing the units of time during which each person in the group was observed. It is expressed as the number of units of 'time at risk', for example 1 person-year = one individual at risk (or observed) for 1 year (or two people for half a year each).

Caution must be exercised in the use of 'time at risk' as a denominator. It is only valid if the risk of developing the disease in an individual is not influenced by the period of exposure or the time at which the exposure occurred. If there is reason to believe that the risk of a disease is affected by the length of time an individual is exposed to an agent, the summation of the exposed time within a group will be misleading. For example, in 1969 Pisciotta demonstrated that chlorpromazine can cause agranulocytosis in some people and that it usually occurs after 5–7 weeks of continuous exposure (Pisciotta AV. *JAMA* 1969; **208**: 1862). It follows that patients who are exposed for less than 5 weeks do not have the same risk as those exposed for longer, even though they might be susceptible. Patients exposed for over 7 weeks clearly have a greatly reduced risk of developing the dyscrasia since they have passed through the critical exposure period. If, in a study designed to assess the risk of agranulocytosis in patients exposed to chlorpromazine, the total number of treatment weeks is used as a denominator, it will give a distorted indication of the level of risk. In this case, the definition of exposure must specify the time period during which the individual consumed the drug.

ADVANTAGES AND DISADVANTAGES OF COHORT STUDIES

Advantages

• The main advantage of the cohort study design is that it is possible to distinguish antecedent causes from concurrent associated factors in the aetiology of disease.

• In both types of cohort study, the incidence of disease in exposed and non-exposed groups can be determined, allowing the calculation of absolute, relative and attributable risks (see p. 14).

• It is possible to study several outcomes from exposure to the same hazard.

• Bias in controls is less of a problem than in case–control studies because the necessary comparison groups (exposed and non-exposed) are built into the study design from the start. Even so, it is important to bear in mind that the two groups may not be equally susceptible to the disease under study.

• Because the study is prospective, it is possible to standardize methods, thereby reducing error due to observer, subject and technical variation (see pp. 42–3).

Disadvantages

• It is not possible to be certain that supposed aetiological factors are in fact causal. This requires experiments of a kind referred to in Chapter 3, which are rarely possible in human populations.

• Even with common diseases, large populations are usually required to obtain significant differences in incidence in exposed and non-exposed groups. Also, if the incubation period of the disease is prolonged, the results of the study may be greatly delayed. These factors tend to make cohort studies very expensive in resources.

• One of the major difficulties encountered in cohort studies is in the follow-up of all subjects. Migration and withdrawal of cooperation may bias the results. It is necessary, therefore, to build into the study design a system for obtaining basic information on the personal characteristics and outcome of those who cannot be followed up in detail for the full duration of the study. This allows comparisons to be made between subjects who are fully studied and those who are not. In this way, serious selective bias may be detected and can be allowed for in the analysis and interpretation of the results.

• Finally, even though standard methods and diagnostic criteria are adopted, these may change owing to 'drift' over a prolonged follow-up period and results in later stages may not be comparable with those obtained earlier in the study.

EXAMPLES OF COHORT STUDIES

Mortality in relation to smoking: 40 years' observations on male British doctors (Doll R, Peto R, Wheatley K, Gray R, Sutherland I. *Br Med J* 1994; **309**: 901–11)

The classic study of the effects of smoking amongst British doctors is a good example of a study based upon a cohort that was used because it was administratively easy to identify and follow-up. It involved the use of an internal control group. In 1951, the research team sent a simple questionnaire to all of the 59 600 doctors whose names were on The Medical Register of the UK at the time. The questionnaire enquired about their past and current smoking habits. Over 34 000 (69%) of the male doctors and more than 6000 (60%) of the female doctors who were contacted completed the questionnaire. The responding doctors were divided according to their past and current smoking habits and their subsequent mortality was recorded. Further questionnaires to obtain information on changes in smoking habits and other data were sent to the male doctors in 1957, 1960, 1972, 1978 and 1990. The fact that all the individuals being studied were doctors on The Medical Register aided follow-up considerably. Deaths of doctors are notified to the Medical Register, for reasons quite unconnected with the study, which enabled the investigators to follow-up a cohort many years after it was recruited with comparative ease. The first stage of the analysis was to divide the doctors into those exposed to the suspected harmful agent (smokers) and those not exposed (non-smokers). The mortality of the two groups was then compared.

The conclusions of the investigators have had far-reaching consequences. An association was found between smoking and seven different cancers, most notably lung cancer, as well as with chronic obstructive lung disease, vascular disease, peptic ulcer and several other fatal diseases. The excess mortality was almost twice as high in the second half of the study as in the first half (Fig. 5.1). It now seems that about half of all regular smokers will eventually be killed by their habit. There was a pronounced correlation between the death rate from lung cancer and the number of cigarettes smoked (Fig. 5.2). The data also revealed that the risk of death from lung cancer fell substantially in those who gave up smoking, a benefit which increased with time.

This study yielded two observations that could not have been made from descriptive studies alone. Firstly, the sequence of events was clearly identified, smoking was followed by lung cancer, and secondly, a dose–response effect was demonstrated. Both of these findings weigh heavily in favour of the causal hypothesis. However, it should be remembered that the investigation was stimulated by the results of descriptive studies which showed a correlation between mortality from lung cancer and sales of cigarettes in England and Wales.

The problem with a cohort recruited in this way is that if it is used to study the effects of an agent or factor which is very rare, or if the disease is a rare consequence of exposure, then the size of the cohort has to be very large in order to yield sufficient numbers of cases to detect a significant difference between the risks in the exposed group and the non-exposed group.

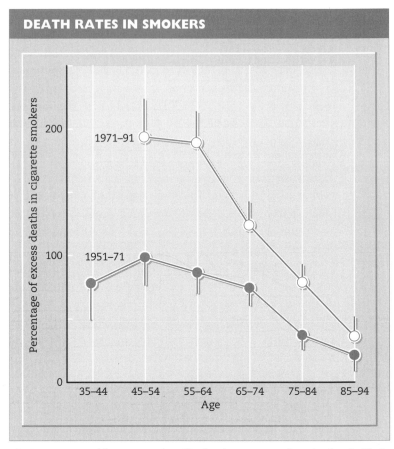

DEATH RATES IN SMOKERS

Fig. 5.1 Age-specific excess mortality in cigarette smokers in first half of study (lower line) contrasted with that in second half (upper line). An excess of 100% represents doubled death rate. Bars indicate standard deviations. (From Doll et al., 1994.)

Survivors of the Hiroshima and Nagasaki atomic explosions

(Brill AB, Masanobu RR, Heyssel RM. *Ann Int Med* 1962; **56**: 590–609)

The second type of cohort, one which is defined by the fact that the individual members have all been exposed to the same experience or agent, has the closest similarity to the laboratory experiment. There are many instances of cohorts that have been defined in this way. For example, the survivors of the atomic bomb explosions in Hiroshima and Nagasaki comprise a unique group of people who were exposed to high levels of ionizing radiation for a short time. In this group of people there was little difficulty in calculating the proportion who developed leukaemia after, say 10 years, i.e. the absolute risk of leukaemia.

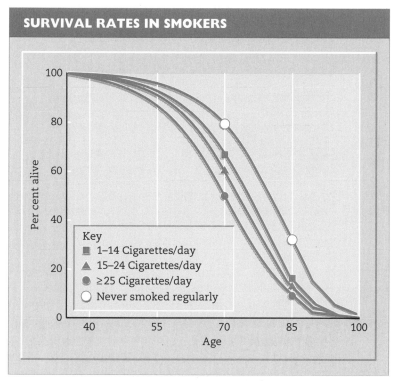

SURVIVAL RATES IN SMOKERS

Key
■ 1–14 Cigarettes/day
▲ 15–24 Cigarettes/day
● ≥25 Cigarettes/day
○ Never smoked regularly

Fig. 5.2 Overall survival after age 35 years among cigarette smokers and non-smokers: life-table estimates, based on specific death rates for the entire 40-year period. (From Doll et al., 1994.)

However, in order to establish whether the incidence of leukaemia in the cohort was more or less than in a group not so exposed – the relative risk of leukaemia – it was necessary to study a group of people who were similar to the exposed group in all respects except for their exposure to ionizing radiation. In one of the many studies of the survivors from Hiroshima and Nagasaki, the control group comprised individuals who were living in the same area but outside the radiation zone. The study showed that the incidence of confirmed leukaemia was between 50 and 100 times greater in the exposed population than in the controls. Further investigations showed a clear relationship between the distance from the epicentre of the explosion and leukaemia incidence rates (Table 5.1), demonstrating a dose–response effect.

Regular fluoroscopy and risk of breast cancer
(Boice JD, Monson RR. *J Nat Cancer Inst* 1977; **59**: 823–32)

A cohort that experienced a different type of ionizing radiation is exem-

NUCLEAR EXPOSURE AND LEUKAEMIA

Distance from epicentre (metres)	Incidence rate per 1 000 000 person-years at risk	
	Hiroshima	Nagasaki
0000–999	1366	563
1000–1499	308	530
1500–1999	42	68
2000–9999	28	37

Table 5.1 Average incidence of confirmed leukaemia in residents of Hiroshima and Nagasaki (1947–58) by city of exposure and distance from epicentre.

plified by the group of people who had large numbers of fluoroscopies in the 1940s and 1950s while being treated for pulmonary tuberculosis before the dangers of X-rays were fully appreciated. It has been shown that young women in the group that were irradiated had a higher than expected incidence of breast cancer. In this study, the control group was all other women of the same age in the population, the great majority of whom, it may be assumed, were not exposed to radiation in this way (Table 5.2).

Social class differences in IHD in men (Pocock SJ, Shaper AG, Cook DG, Phillips AN, Walker M. *Lancet* 1987; **ii**: 197–201)

During 1979–80, 7735 men aged 40–59 years were randomly selected from the 'lists' of people registered with general practitioners in 24 towns in England, Scotland and Wales and were asked to participate in a long-term study. Seventy-eight per cent of those who were approached agreed to cooperate. These men were asked to complete a questionnaire which included questions on occupation, smoking habits and indicators of heart disease. They were also examined by a research nurse. Ninety-nine per cent of the men were followed up for an average of 6 years.

The data were analysed using a multiple logistic regression model in order to adjust simultaneously the incidence rates of major IHD events for smoking, systolic blood pressure, serum cholesterol, age and social class.

Of these men, 336 experienced major IHD events (defined as fatal IHD or myocardial infarction). The crude attack rates and the attack rates adjusted for the risk factors set out above are shown in Table 5.3.

FLUOROSCOPY AND BREAST CANCER	
Age at first exposure (years)	Relative risk
<15	2.1
15–19	3.8
20–24	1.7
25–29	1.6
30–34	1.2
35–39	0.8
40+	0.9

Table 5.2 Relative risk of breast cancer in women subjected to regular fluoroscopies at different ages (risk in general population = 1).

SOCIAL CLASS AND IHD			
		Cases per 1000 per annum	
Social class category	Number of IHD cases	Adjusted	Unadjusted
I	21	5.6 ⎫	7.4 ⎫
II	56	5.2 ⎬ 5.5	6.0 ⎬ 6.0
III non-manual	27	6.0 ⎭	6.0 ⎭
III manual	169	8.2 ⎫	7.7 ⎫
IV	36	7.4 ⎬ 7.9	7.3 ⎬ 7.5
V	11	5.6 ⎭	5.0 ⎭

Table 5.3 Attack rates of major IHD events during follow-up, before and after adjustment for social class differences in risk factors.

The results indicate that, after taking account of the differences in smoking habits, systolic blood pressure, serum cholesterol and age between the social class groups, there remains an unexplained higher incidence of major IHD events amongst men in manual occupations compared to those in non-manual occupations.

CHAPTER 6

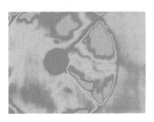

Case–Control Studies

INTRODUCTION

Case–control studies are often used for the preliminary investigation of a hypothesis, and may be followed by cohort and/or intervention studies to explore and test the hypothesis more fully. They enquire into events that occurred before recruitment to the study and usually before the onset of illness in cases of the disease. They are therefore sometimes called retrospective studies. They involve comparing individuals who are identified because they are known to have the disease (cases) with individuals who do not have the disease being investigated (controls). The past histories and exposures to suspected harmful agents of cases and controls are ascertained either by direct questioning or by reference to their clinical or other records. The frequencies with which the same characteristics or exposures are found in the two groups are compared. The simplest comparisons are of the frequency rates of the antecedent factors between groups. Thereafter it may be profitable to use more complex statistical techniques that take account of more than one variable at a time to investigate their relative importance. A greater frequency of a factor under investigation in the diseased group lends support to an aetiological hypothesis, but it will not necessarily prove causation. This is because the sequence of events is not always clear. For example, if men with coronary heart disease are found to follow a sedentary occupation more often than controls, it is not clear whether lack of exercise predisposes to heart disease or whether those with incipient cardiac problems choose less physically demanding jobs.

SELECTION OF CASES

The value of a case–control study is profoundly influenced by the ways in which both the cases and the controls are selected. Ideally, all the cases of the disease in a defined population should be included in the investigation. However, it is rarely feasible or indeed necessary to do this in order to reach sensible and valid conclusions. Most studies are implicitly or explicitly concerned with a sample of cases, usually identified by some form of cluster sampling technique (see p. 40). The 'cluster' used will depend upon the disease that is being investigated and the availability and accessibility of information about patients who are affected by the disease. Sources that are commonly used to identify cases include hospital in-patients, patients attending hospital out-patient departments or their general practitioner, patients who are on disease registers such as cancer registers, and death certificates. Whatever the source that is used, it is important to establish that all people with the disease have an equal chance of being identified through that source if it is intended to extrapolate the findings of the study beyond the circumstances in which it was undertaken.

These principles can be illustrated by considering the selection of cases for a study of risk factors associated with carcinoma of the breast. It would be reasonable to recruit the cases from amongst women being treated in hospital for the first time for breast cancer, as there is a high probability that all cases of breast cancer will receive hospital treatment or hospital care before they die, and without treatment the disease is nearly always fatal. By contrast, the identification of cases for a study of peptic ulcer is more difficult since not all people with peptic ulceration seek medical help for their condition. The identification of cases at a source of medical care may introduce bias into the investigation because the factors that lead an individual to seek attention are not necessarily related either to the severity of the disease or its symptoms. In effect, patients who seek medical attention for a peptic ulcer, whether at hospital or in general practice, are unlikely to be a random sample of individuals affected with a peptic ulcer. The more specialized the source of these patients, for example gastroenterology in-patients, the more selective is the group, and consequently general conclusions from the results of the study become less secure. In situations such as this it is often necessary to conduct a prevalence survey in a general population (see p. 37) in order to identify cases for inclusion in a study.

Once the appropriate source of patients for study has been identified—

the cluster—the same principles of sampling from the cluster can be applied as have been explained in Chapter 4.

SELECTION OF CONTROLS

Control subjects are essential in order to establish the frequency with which the suspected causal agents or determinants occur in people who do not have the disease under investigation. Controls should be a representative sample of the population from which the cases were recruited and thus are at similar risk of having been exposed to the suspected agent. Once selected, controls should neither be discarded nor replaced for any reason other than that they fail to meet the selection criteria, for example if they were mistakenly drawn from another population.

The similarity between controls and cases in relevant characteristics can be ensured by selecting controls individually to match cases by appropriate criteria, for example age, sex and any other variable which may affect the risk of exposure to an agent or risk of contracting disease but which is not one of the variables under study. These are called matched pairs. The limitation of using this method of selection is that the effects of the characteristics which form the basis of the matching cannot always be known in advance and there is a danger that over-rigorous matching may lead to failure to identify a significant variable. Alternatively, matching may be on a group basis, i.e. selection of controls at random from a sample of the parent population from which the cases were drawn. Sometimes, in order to increase statistical sensitivity in the analysis of the results, more than one control is selected for each case, particularly if the number of cases is small. Data must be obtained and observations made in a precisely similar manner for controls as for cases.

It is important to note that error (or bias) in the selection of controls will have exactly the same effect on the outcome of the study as bias in the selection of cases. In case–control studies (and in cohort studies that involve selection of external controls) as much attention must be given to the identification of, and collection of data from, the control subjects as is given to the cases.

The following are examples of groups from which control subjects can be recruited.
• People working in the same factory or attending the same school or living in the same locality as cases.
• Routine registers such as birth registers, electoral rolls, payrolls, school rolls or practice lists. Each of these potentially has its own selective bias which must be recognized in making a choice.

• Hospital patients, either all attenders or, more usually, those with conditions believed to be unrelated to the factors under study. The main limitation of using hospital patients as controls in any study is that, even though they may not have the disease being investigated, they are unlikely to be a random sample of the general population from which the cases are drawn. For example, even though a hospital patient does not have the disease under investigation he or she may have another disease caused by the same agent or whose presence could have affected exposure to the causal agent of the disease under investigation. Moreover, people who live in poor social environments are more likely to be admitted to hospital than those who live in better circumstances and their use as controls may introduce a social class bias.

• Relatives and spouses. These have the advantages of accessibility and willingness to cooperate, ease of location and of sharing the same environmental conditions. Obviously they are unsuitable where genetic or home environment factors are under study. It is also unlikely that such a selection process will result in the same sex ratio as the cases unless the occurrence of the disease is unrelated to sex.

• Control subjects for some case–control studies have been identified through random digit dialling using telephone exchanges serving the areas in which the cases are resident. Using this method, controls that fail to meet basic recruitment criteria are discarded after a few key questions and the remainder are included in the investigation.

RISK IN COHORT AND CASE–CONTROL STUDIES

Cohort studies are designed to provide the data needed to calculate incidence rates of the disease amongst individuals exposed to the suspected causal agent and those not exposed. By contrast, case–control studies only provide data from which the rate of exposure to suspected harmful agents in diseased and non-diseased individuals can be calculated. This means that neither the absolute nor the attributable risk or precise relative risk resulting from exposure can be calculated. The difficulty is shown schematically in Tables 6.1 and 6.2.

In a cohort study, the subjects studied are all those exposed $(A + C)$ and all those not exposed $(B + D)$ to the suspected causal agent (Table 6.1). The subjects subsequently reveal themselves as diseased or non-diseased within these categories. There is, therefore, no difficulty in calculating the disease rate in the total population $(A + B/A + B + C + D)$ or in the exposed persons $(A/(A + C))$ and those not exposed $(B/B + D))$.

COHORT STUDIES			
	Disease present	Disease absent	Total
Exposed to suspected cause	A	C	A + C
Not exposed to suspected cause	B	D	B + D
Total	A + B	C + D	A + B + C + D

Table 6.1 Information available in cohort studies.

CASE–CONTROL STUDY		
	Diseased	Not diseased
Suspected cause present	a	c
Suspected cause absent	b	d
Total	a + b	c + d

Table 6.2 Division of subjects in a case–control study.

The subsequent calculation of relative risk (RR) and attributable risk (AR) presents no problem:

$$RR = \frac{A}{A+C} \text{ divided by } \frac{B}{B+D} = \frac{A \times (B+D)}{B \times (A+C)}$$

$$AR = \frac{A}{A+C} \text{ minus } \frac{B}{B+D}$$

The subjects in a case–control study are identified either because they have the disease (the cases) or because they do not have the disease (the controls) that is being investigated. They are subsequently sub-divided into 'exposed' and 'not exposed' sub-groups (Table 6.2). It is not possible to derive the total numbers of cases in the population who were exposed and not exposed because a case–control study is not based upon a known proportion of the population in either category. Consequently, neither the incidence rate in the population as a whole nor the incidence rate amongst the people exposed to the suspected harmful agent can be derived. It follows from this that risk cannot be calculated directly. However, an approximation of the relative risk can be derived from case–control data. This approximation, although often referred to as the relative risk, is more correctly termed the odds ratio (OR). It is calculated as follows. Using the notation in Table 6.1 the true relative risk is:

$$\frac{A \times (B+D)}{B \times (A+C)}$$

In the case of most diseases, the proportion of the population who are affected, whether or not they are exposed to the suspected causal agent, is small. Thus, A is small in relation to C; likewise B is small in relation to D. It follows that D will approximate to B + D and C will approximate to A + C. The approximation to the relative risk, the OR, then becomes:

$$\frac{A \times D}{B \times C} = \frac{a \times d}{b \times c}$$

This approximation to relative risk is used in all case–control studies but it is only valid if the incidence of the disease is low. In most circumstances it is not possible to calculate attributable risk from a case–control study.

ADJUSTING FOR CONFOUNDING VARIABLES

There are two ways to take account of confounding variables.

1 *Analysis of sub-sets of the data to adjust for the confounding variable.* This can be illustrated by considering a study of the effect of age at first birth on womens' risk of carcinoma of the breast. Women who have their first child whilst young tend to have more children than women whose first child is born late in their reproductive life. It follows that if there is a statistical association between age at first birth and the risk of breast cancer it is likely that there will also be an association between family size and risk of breast cancer. The two effects can be separated by restricting the analysis to women who have had only one child (thereby separating out the effects of parity) and calculating the risk according to age at first pregnancy. Or the analysis can be restricted to women who had their first child at a given age and calculating the risks according to parity. The disadvantage of this technique is that not all the available data can be used in the critical analyses.

2 *Use of a multivariate analysis technique to adjust the relative risk for the effect of confounding variables.* The advent of accessible and powerful computing has made it possible to use highly sophisticated mathematical techniques to analyse data from epidemiological studies. The calculation of an adjusted relative risk using logistic regression is one such technique. An advantage of this method is that it allows simultaneous adjustment for

the effects of more than one confounding variable. Similar methods are used to adjust for the effects of confounding variables in cohort studies. A discussion of the mathematics of this method is beyond the scope of this text; it is considered by Armitage and Berry (see Appendix).

EFFECTS OF HIGH INCIDENCE OF EXPOSURE

Essentially, the success of a case–control study is dependent upon there being a significant difference between the proportion of cases exposed to the suspect agent and the number of controls so exposed. If the incidence of exposure is very high, it may be impossible to demonstrate such a difference. Consider an extreme example of a case–control study designed to identify the possible causal agents of carcinoma of the bronchus which is conducted in a population where the prevalence of cigarette smoking over the age of 15 years is 100%. In such a situation there can be no difference between the proportion of cases and controls exposed to cigarettes. It follows that smoking could not be revealed as a risk factor. It does not follow that no risk factors will be revealed by such a study, but those identified may be associated rather than causal and the principal cause will be missed.

ADVANTAGES AND DISADVANTAGES OF CASE–CONTROL STUDIES

Advantages

Despite the approximations that have to be made in the analysis of case–control studies, they do have some important advantages over cohort studies.
• By concentrating effort on the identification of affected individuals and recruiting controls from the unaffected population, the number of subjects required to obtain significant results is kept to a minimum.
• Results can be obtained relatively quickly because the investigation does not have to wait for the disease to develop, as it does in cohort studies. This means that it is a relatively inexpensive type of study.

Disadvantages

• Case–control studies generally rely upon retrospective data, which have their own inherent problems. The ability of individuals to recall past events tends to be unreliable due to a tendency for memory to be selective. Records of past events may be incomplete in respect of variables that are the subject of investigation, and the ways in which the relevant observations and measurements were made are not usually standardized. This gives rise to uncertainty regarding their validity.

• Because the data are collected after the event (retrospectively) it is difficult to be sure whether a demonstrable correlation is causal or not. Thus, the finding that a history of cigarette smoking is common amongst individuals with lung cancer does not prove that the former preceded and caused the latter. Alternative explanations are that people who choose to smoke are also constitutionally predisposed to long cancer or are exposed to another noxious agent more often than are non-smokers. This problem is less conspicuous when dealing with highly specific agents such as micro-organisms or in situations where the time between exposure and onset of symptoms is short.

• There are sometimes difficulties in selecting and recruiting appropriate controls. This is important because the value of the results obtained from a case–control study is as dependent upon the proper selection of 'controls' as it is on the identification of affected individuals.

• Because case–control studies are not based on defined populations, the incidence of the disease within that population cannot be calculated from the study.

EXAMPLES OF CASE–CONTROL STUDIES

Sexual activity, contraceptive method, genital infections and cervical cancer (Slattery M, Overall JC, Abbott TM et al. Am J Epidemiol 1989; **130**: 248–58)

It has been suggested that cervical cancer is a sexually transmitted disease. Between 1984 and 1987 a case–control study was carried out in Utah, USA, where a high proportion of the population are active members of the Church of Jesus Christ of Latter Day Saints (Mormons). The study was designed to explore the relationship between cervical cancer and sexual activity, the use of barrier methods of contraception and certain types of genital infection. The subjects were women aged 20–59 years, newly diagnosed with cervical cancer. Controls were identified by use of a random digit-dialling telephone sampling technique. They were matched to cases by 5-year age intervals and county of residence. Interviews were completed for 266 women with histologically confirmed carcinoma-*in-situ* or invasive squamous cell cervical cancer and for 408 matched controls.

After adjustment for age, education, church attendance and cigarette

CERVICAL CANCER AND RISK

Risk factor	Numbers		Odds ratio	
	Cases	Controls	Crude	Adjusted
Number of sex partners of woman				
<2	25	210	1.00	1.00
2–3	54	73	6.21	3.43
4–5	47	53	7.44	3.59
6–10	57	39	12.27	5.51
>10	69	28	20.70	8.99
Number of sex partners of mate				
1	24	198	1.00	1.00
2–3	42	78	4.44	2.72
4–5	38	39	8.03	4.99
6–10	45	22	16.87	7.98
>10	49	23	17.57	2.10
Trichomonas infections	53	21	4.61	2.10
Herpes type 2 (neutralization index >1000)	12	6	6.57	2.70

Table 6.3 Risk factors for cervical cancer.

smoking, by means of multiple logistic regression models, several significant risk factors were identified. These included multiple sex partners, current mate having multiple sex partners, reported *Trichomonas* infection and serological evidence of herpes virus type 2 infection (Table 6.3). It should be noted that there is a pronounced gradient of risk relating to increased numbers of partners and increased numbers of partners of the mate of the woman.

A protective effect was noted from use of foam or jelly as a contraceptive method (OR = 0.44), from the use of diaphragms (OR = 0.67) or condoms (OR = 0.53), in women who reported more than one sex partner. These data lend support to the hypothesis that cervical cancer is due to a sexually transmitted agent.

Pertussis immunization and serious acute neurological illnesses in children (Miller DL, Madge N, Diamond J, Wadsworth J, Ross EM. *Br Med J* 1993; **307**: 1171–6)

In 1975, widespread public alarm was created by the suggestion that whooping cough vaccine might cause severe encephalopathic illnesses followed by permanent brain damage in a small but significant number of children. It would have been impractical and unethical to conduct a large-scale randomized control trial to test the validity of this suggestion. Therefore, a case–control study was set up which aimed to identify all children admitted to hospitals in the UK with serious acute neurological illnesses of the types which it was suggested could be caused by the vaccine and lead to permanent brain damage. For each case child reported, two control children, matched for age and sex, were selected from those living in the same local area. The past histories of immunization and of other possible predisposing or aetiological factors were obtained for both case and control children in identical manners. Of 904 cases of encephalopathy and severe convulsions reported, 30 (3.3%) had received pertussis vaccine within 7 days before becoming ill, compared with 23 (1.3%) of 1783 control children immunized within 7 days before a defined reference date, which was a significant difference (OR = 3.3) (Table 6.4). The children were followed up a decade later to determine the late outcome of their illnesses. Nearly two-thirds had either died or were suffering from significant neurological dysfunction. Of 367 such children, 12 (3.3%) were pertussis vaccine-associated compared with 6 (0.8%) of 723 controls, which gives an OR of 5.5. Thus, the study showed that there is a small but definite risk of serious acute neurological illnesses after whooping cough vaccine, though the risk was much smaller than some workers had suggested from totally uncontrolled series of cases. It was also clear that children who suffered from such illnesses often died or had significant long-term sequelae, though the number of such cases associated with recent pertussis immunization was too small to be certain that the vaccine was on its own responsible for cases of permanent brain

ENCEPHALOPATHY				
	All outcomes		Dead or dysfunction 10 years later	
	n	Vaccine associated (%)	n	Vaccine associated (%)
Cases	904	30 (3.3)	367	12 (3.3)
Controls	1783	23 (1.3)	723	6 (0.8)
OR		3.3		5.5

Table 6.4 Pertussis vaccine and encephalopathy in children.

damage. This study illustrates the difficulty of identifying aetiological factors in extremely rare conditions.

Perinatal deaths and maternal occupation (Clarke M, Mason ES. Br Med J 1985; **290**: 1235–7)

Reproductive hazards are thought to exist in many industries. In order to explore this problem, a case–control study of perinatal death occurring in Leicestershire was carried out between 1976 and 1982. Case notes were reviewed and the mothers were interviewed in all 1187 cases of perinatal death during this period. The control for each case was selected as the next live birth occurring at the place, or intended place of delivery. All maternal and paternal occupations and industries were recorded at the interview with the mother. A total of 671 mothers were employed outside the home at some time during pregnancy. An analysis of maternal occupations showed that the OR for the risk of perinatal death was exceptionally high in women employed in the leather industry (OR = 2.1 after adjustment for social class). A similar excess was found in all towns within the county where shoe manufacture took place. No other risk factor was found to account for this observation. Possible hazards appeared to be the leather, or adhesives used, or both. Further studies will be required to identify the specifc hazardous exposure in these women.

Results of case–control study of leukaemia and lymphoma among young people near Sellafield nuclear plant in West Cumbria (Gardner MJ, Snee MP, Hall AJ, Powell CA, Downes S, Terrell JD. Br Med J 1990; **300**: 423–9)

Concern about levels of childhood cancers around nuclear installations and a consequent public enquiry led to several studies being set up. One was a case–control study of leukaemia and lymphoma among young people living in the vicinity of the Sellafield nuclear plant in West Cumbria. Its aims were to explore whether known causes or factors associated with the nuclear site were responsible for the apparent excess. A total of 74 cases of leukaemia and lymphoma among people born in West Cumbria and diagnosed there at ages under 25 between 1950 and 1985 was identified. Risk factors in cases were compared with those in up to eight controls matched by date of birth and sex, selected from the same birth register as their respective cases. The expected association with prenatal exposure to X-rays was found, but the main finding was of significantly raised relative risks in children born near Sellafield and in children whose fathers were employed at the plant (RR = 2.4), particularly those fathers with high radiation-dose recordings before the child's conception (RR = 6.4). At the time, no other satisfactory explanation was put forward and it was concluded that ionizing radiation may be leukaemogenic to offspring. This interpretation has been subsequently challenged in the scientific literature.

CHAPTER 7

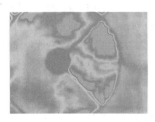

Intervention Studies

INTRODUCTION

Descriptive, cohort and case–control studies are used to develop and test hypotheses about the possible causes and determinants of disease. The results may suggest methods of prevention or treatment which then need to be formally evaluated. Intervention studies are most often used for this purpose and are commonly called clinical trials. They are essentially experimental studies in which the efficacy and safety of medical management of disease is evaluated by comparing the outcome of the intervention in test and control groups. The intervention under test is most often a new preventive or treatment regime, but the method can also be used to compare different established regimes and to evaluate the effectiveness and efficiency of different forms of service provision. Experimental studies in which the incidence of a disease in those deliberately exposed to a suspected causal agent, or protected from it, is compared with that in controls can also be of value and provide the most convincing evidence of a causal relationship. However, for practical and ethical reasons this approach is rarely adopted except in animal studies.

METHODS IN CLINICAL TRIALS

The methodologies of preventive and therapeutic trials have some similarities to those used in cohort studies. The basis of a clinical trial is the random allocation of individuals in a population to 'test' and 'control' groups. The intervention measure under trial is applied to the test group but not to the control group and the effect is assessed in terms of the same defined outcome in both groups. The particular form of intervention whose effects are being tested is called the independent variable, while the outcome being measured is called the dependent variable. The selection of the study population should be governed by the following considerations.

• The population under study should be representative of the population in which it is intended to apply the intervention being tested (this is called the target population).

• It is important to choose a stable population in which there are unlikely to be heavy losses during the follow-up period and whose cooperation is reasonably assured. Volunteers are usually not acceptable since they tend to differ from non-volunteers in important respects, such as motivation and past history of illness.

• The likely frequency of the outcome being measured should be known, since this critically affects the required sample size. It is usually convenient to choose a group with a high incidence of the outcome being investigated in order to economize on numbers.

• The population should be readily accessible. Trials are often most conveniently conducted in patients attending general practice or hospital, in residential institutions, factories, the armed forces, etc., even though they may not fairly represent the general population in all respects.

ALLOCATION TO TEST AND CONTROL GROUPS

In principle, the allocation of patients to test and control groups should be random, hence the term sometimes applied to clinical trials, randomized controlled trials (RCTs). The aim is to ensure that those treated and those untreated are exactly similar in all respects prior to intervention. This is necessary to guard against the possibility that some factor other than the intervention could account for differences in outcome in the two groups.

TYPES OF RANDOM ALLOCATION

• Individual: by date of birth etc.
• Cluster: of whole groups or communities
• Stratified: random selection within specified sub-groups
• No allocation: for ethical reasons, e.g. new vaccine trials in children

Individual allocation

The allocation of individuals to test or control groups can be by day of birth, registration number or other suitable procedure. This is the usual method adopted in clinical trials. Alternate allocation to test and control is to be avoided, as it may enable the patient or the person who assesses the outcome to guess the group to which the subject has been allocated.

Cluster allocation

For practical reasons, allocation is sometimes made of whole groups or communities. This is because, for example in trials of a vaccine, the spread of infection may be inhibited in unvaccinated people if a propor-tion of the population is protected, thereby obscuring the benefit derived from vaccination. Similarly, in recent trials of preventive advice against coronary heart disease, the test and control groups were workers in randomly allocated factories, in order to minimize 'contamination' of the control group with advice offered to the intervention group.

Stratified allocation

Where the population is relatively small and non-homogeneous, random selection within specified sub-groups, for example age groups, may be desirable to ensure similarity in relevant characteristics between test and control groups.

No allocation

Sometimes random allocation of treatment would not be ethical, for example a trial of a new type of measles vaccine in children. In this case, the comparison must be with past experience or that in other populations. It is difficult in such cases to measure the extent of any benefit with confidence.

Since willingness to cooperate may not be randomly distributed in the population, allocation should be deferred until agreement to participate has been obtained.

To avoid bias in reporting illnesses and other possible behavioural differences, subjects should not know to which group they have been allocated. In drug and vaccine trials, this often entails the use of a placebo treatment for controls which must be presented in an identical form to the active treatment. In the case of some procedures, for example provision of different types of service, blind allocation is not possible. A trial in which neither the subject nor the people assessing outcome know whether the subject is receiving active treatment or not (or which of two different treatments is being given) is called a double-blind trial.

OUTCOME (DEPENDENT VARIABLE)

The outcome to be assessed must be specified in advance. It should be expressed in terms of advantage to the patient or to the community, for example reduced incidence or severity of disease or cost to the health service. Assessment criteria should be clearly defined, consistently applied and reliably recorded in order to minimize bias in the measurement of outcome. Misclassified cases in either test or control group will reduce the size of difference between them in the incidence of disease and thus give a spuriously reduced apparent benefit from the treatment. The safety of an intervention is as important as its efficacy and the assessment of outcome should always include the frequency of adverse effects of the intervention as well as its benefits.

FOLLOW-UP

Procedures for the follow-up of subjects in both test and control groups should be the same, giving particular attention to the following.

• The data collected must be obtained and recorded in a standard manner.

• The method used should be simple and should be sufficiently sensitive to detect reliably all relevant events in members of the study population.

• Follow-up must be equally rigorous in both test and control groups.

• Follow-up must start from the time of allocation and continue for long enough to evaluate fully the outcome in all subjects.

• Cooperation must be maintained at the highest possible level, and losses from the study population for any reasons should be minimized.

ANALYSIS

The efficacy of an intervention is usually measured as the proportion of the expected incidence which is prevented by the intervention expressed as a percentage, i.e.

$$\frac{[\text{expected incidence (controls)} - \text{intervention incidence (test)}] \times 100}{\text{expected incidence}}$$

For example, in a vaccine trial:

incidence in vaccinated children = 5 per 1000
incidence in unvaccinated children = 50 per 1000

$$\text{efficacy} = \frac{50 - 5}{50} = \frac{45}{50} = 90\%$$

SEQUENTIAL ANALYSIS

Sometimes, when a result is required urgently or when the anticipated benefits are high or the possible adverse effects are serious, the results are analysed sequentially. This technique involves continuous data analysis and allows the trial to be stopped immediately when a significantly beneficial or adverse effect has been demonstrated or when the results fail to reach a previously defined level of significance, usually that which the investigators regard as the minimum useful benefit.

ETHICAL CONSIDERATIONS

The ethical questions that arise in the planning and conduct of RCTs are shown below.

ETHICS

- What are the possible risks of treatment and of failure to treat?
- Is it right to expose some people to possible harm from an untested treatment or to withhold from others a possibly beneficial treatment?
- Is it right to introduce a new treatment into use without first assessing its safety and benefits by a properly conducted trial?
- To what extent should a trial be explained to the subjects before they agree to participate?
- How can the welfare and safety of participants be safeguarded while preserving the principle of 'blind' assessment?

In general, it is best to carry out a trial before a new treatment is accepted into routine practice. Usually potent new drugs and vaccines are in short supply initially and it is impossible to offer them to everyone. At this stage, random allocation of patients to the new treatment in a properly conducted trial may be as fair a means of selection as any, and full advantage should be taken of the opportunity. Where omission of active treatment or giving a placebo may be dangerous, the controls are often given conventional treatment. In this case, the aim is to measure the additional advantage from the new treatment.

The MRC, the WHO and others have issued guidelines for resolving some of the ethical problems of clinical trials. Health districts and research institutions now have 'Ethical Committees' with both broad professional and lay representation. These offer research workers the benefit of advice from a group of uncommitted individuals who can review the protocol dispassionately, though final responsibility must always rest with the scientist doing the work.

EXAMPLES OF INTERVENTION STUDIES

MRC trial of treatment of mild hypertension
(Medical Research Council Working Party. *Br Med J* 1985; **291**: 97–104)

It has long been known that people with high blood pressure have an increased risk of stroke and other cardiovascular events and that treatment is effective in reducing the incidence of these conditions in severe hypertension. However, the value of treating mild hypertension compared with disadvantages of long-term therapy in otherwise healthy people was less certain. An RCT of treatment in such cases was therefore carried out by the MRC. Even though hypertension and cardiovascular complications are relatively common conditions, it was calculated that this would require a very large-scale trial in order to obtain a statistically significant result. Subjects for the trial were found by screening blood pressure measurements in 515000 people aged 35–64 years selected from the age–sex registers of 176 general practices in England, Scotland and Wales.

In this way 17354 patients with a diastolic pressure in the range 90–109 mmHg and systolic pressure below 200 mmHg were identified. Patients were randomly allocated to one of four groups, two of which were treated with different hypotensive drugs and two with placebo tablets which looked identical to the active drug tablets. Randomization was stratified by age and sex. The target level of blood pressure was below 90 mmHg to be reached within 6 months of entry. The study was single-blind only, i.e. the doctor knew the treatment group to which the patients were allocated, but the patients did not. This was to enable the doctor to adjust drug dosage in those on active treatment if necessary to achieve the target level of blood pressure. All other management was the same in both treatment and placebo groups. Recruiting took place over 9 years and the data were analysed sequentially every 6 months in order

MILD HYPERTENSION

Event	Active treatment		Placebo		Percentage difference
	Number	Rate	Number	Rate	
Stroke	60	1.4	109	2.6	45
Coronary events	222	5.4	234	5.5	6
All cardiovascular events	286	6.7	352	8.2	19
All cardiovascular deaths	134	3.1	139	3.3	4
Non-cardiovascular deaths	114	2.7	114	2.7	0

Table 7.1 Mild hypertension: main events in treatment and control groups.

to test whether any significant differences were emerging. In the end, 85 572 person-years of observation accrued. There was a very significant reduction in the incidence of stroke in the treated group, but no difference in the rates of coronary events (Table 7.1). The overall incidence of cardiovascular events was reduced, but mortality from these and all causes was not. It was concluded that if 850 mildly hypertensive patients are given treatment for a year, about one stroke will be prevented. On the other hand, this would subject a substantial percentage of patients to chronic side effects, most but not all of which would be minor.

Prevention of rickets in Asian children: assessment of the Glasgow campaign (Dunnigan MG, Glekin BM, Henderson JB et al. Br Med J 1985; 291: 239–42)

There have been many reports of vitamin D deficiency leading to rickets in infants and school children, and osteomalacia in women among the British Asian community. Theoretically, this would be easily remedied. The treatment is clear cut and no trial of the efficacy of vitamin D is needed. The acceptability of a prophylactic programme and its effectiveness in reducing the prevalence of rickets, however, needed to be assessed. Random allocation of individuals to treatment and control groups would be inappropriate and unethical and, in such circumstances, though less than ideal, a before-and-after intervention assessment is often used. This study reported on the results of a campaign to promote the use of vitamin D supplementation in Glasgow. In a precampaign survey, blood samples were obtained from 189 children aged 5–17 years and those with biochemical evidence of rickets had an X-ray examination of the knees. In postcampaign surveys, 2 and 3 years later, 255 children were similarly examined. On both occasions the children were asked about their frequency of consumption of vitamin D supplements (in younger children this was checked with mothers). The results showed a striking reduction in the prevalence of rickets in children who took regular or even intermittent vitamin D supplements, and the number of hospital discharges of Asian children with rickets in Glasgow declined rapidly after the start of the campaign.

Clearly, the decline in rickets could have been due to factors other than the official vitamin D supplement campaign, for example increasing adoption of a Western diet and lifestyle. However, the time and place reduction in rickets prevalence, backed by objective measures, lends support to an assessment of the effectiveness of the campaign.

RCT of anti-smoking advice: final 20 year results
(Rose G, Colwell L. *J Epidemiol Community Health* 1992; **46**: 75–7)

Many studies have shown that the mortality and morbidity of ex-smokers is less than that of those who continue to smoke. On this basis, smokers are confidently advised to give up smoking in the expectation that their health and prognosis will improve. However, ex-smokers are not a random sample of former smokers and their reasons for giving up may be related to other factors which influence their risk of developing smoking-related diseases. Nor is it certain how effective anti-smoking advice is in influencing smoking behaviour. Therefore, in 1968 the authors set up an RCT of anti-smoking advice in 1445 male smokers, aged 40–59 years, at high risk of developing cardiorespiratory disease. They were allocated at random to an 'intervention' group who were given individual advice on the relationship of smoking to health and challenged to consider their situation. Those who declared a wish to stop smoking were given support and encouragement for an average of four further visits over 12 months. The 'control' group were given no specific advice. All subjects completed a questionnaire 1, 3 and 9 years later. Deaths in the group were monitored. After 1 year, the reported cigarette consumption in the intervention group was one-quarter of that in the control group and over 10 years the net reported reduction averaged 53%. However, the 'normal-care' group also reduced their consumption reflecting a general decline in smoking in the population, thereby reducing the apparent benefit of smoking cessation in the intervention group over the ensuing years. Over the first 10 years, the intervention group experienced fewer respiratory symptoms and less loss of ventilatory function, their mortality from coronary heart disease was 18% lower than controls, and for lung cancer it was 23% lower. No further contact with subjects to determine changes in smoking habits has been attempted, but follow-up has been continued for a further 10 years based on death certificates and cancer registrations. Comparing the intervention with the normal-care group, total mortality was 7% lower, fatal coronary heart disease was 13% lower and lung cancer cases (deaths and registrations) were 11% lower. It was concluded that the policy of encouraging smokers to give up the habit was worthwhile and should not be changed. It was estimated that out of every 100 men who stopped smoking, between 6 and 10 were in consequence alive 20 years later.

Prevention of neural tube defects: results of the MRC Vitamin Study (MRC Vitamin Study Research Group. *Lancet* 1991; **338**: 131–7)

It has long been suspected that diet has a role in the causation of neural tube defects, one of the commonest severe congenital malformations. The possibility that supplementation with folic acid or other vitamins might reduce the risks was given credence by the results of two intervention studies, both of which had methodological weaknesses. A large RCT was needed to resolve the matter. The trial was conducted in 33 centres in seven countries amongst 1817 women known to be at high risk through having had a previous affected pregnancy. They were allocated at random to one of four groups who received supplementation with folic acid and/or other vitamins or none. Of 27 babies born to these women with a neural tube defect, six were in the group who received folic acid supplementation and 21 in the other two groups – a 72% protective effect (RR = 0.28) (Table 7.2). The other vitamins showed no benefit. It was concluded that folic acid supplementation starting before pregnancy can now be firmly recommended for all women who have had an affected pregnancy. There are also grounds for public health action to ensure that the diet of all women who may bear children contains an adequate amount of folic acid.

NEURAL TUBE DEFECTS AND VITAMINS			
Folic acid	Other vitamins	NTD/all babies	RR
+	–	2/298 ⎫ 6/593 (1.0%)	
+	+	4/295 ⎭	
			0.28
–	–	13/300 ⎫ 21/602 (3.5%)	
–	+	8/302 ⎭	

Table 7.2 Neural tube defects (NTD) and folic acid supplementation.

CHAPTER 8

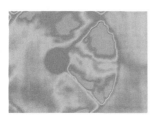

Health Information and Sources of Data

INTRODUCTION

Health is an elusive concept. The WHO has defined it as 'a state of complete physical, mental and social wellbeing'. It is, however, difficult if not impossible to use this definition to measure the health of populations in any categorical sense. Its principal limitation is that an individual's sense of 'wellbeing' is intimately related to that person's expectations from life; these are difficult to measure objectively. Therefore, in order to measure and compare the health of populations, there are few alternatives other than to make use of indices of death and disease, despite the fact that these are the antithesis of health. The calculation of death rates and disease rates requires both numerator data about the events being studied (death and disease) and denominator data about the populations in which the events take place.

This chapter is concerned with routinely collected data used in the measurement of health, mainly from official sources.

CENSUS DATA

Most developed countries undertake regular and detailed censuses of their populations in order to provide information to assist in social and fiscal planning. Although there is evidence that many of the ancient empires, for example Babylon and Egypt, undertook occasional, quite sophisticated censuses, it was the Romans who introduced it as a regular administrative exercise. They did this primarily for taxation assessment purposes. Perhaps the most famous Roman census was the one which took the parents of Christ to Bethlehem at the time of his birth. After the fall of the Roman Empire, the regular counting of populations ceased. In England, the first post-Roman attempt to enumerate the population resulted in the compilation of the Domesday Book in the eleventh century. In common with most of their predecessors, the administrators at that time were concerned to identify families rather than individuals, and even families of different status were recorded differently. From the material that survives, it is not possible to derive a precise figure of the population at that time.

The modern system of censuses was introduced in Europe during the late eighteenth and early nineteenth centuries. In England and Wales, the first complete census was undertaken at the behest of Parliament in 1801. Since then there has been a full census every 10 years, with the exception of 1941. In recent years, 10% sample censuses have been undertaken midway between the full decennial censuses. The census is conducted by the OPCS, a government department. Each census is undertaken only with the specific authority of Parliament. Any individual who refuses to cooperate is liable to prosecution.

The precise information that is collected varies from census to census but it invariably includes age, sex, marital condition, place of birth, occupation, number of children, usual place of residence and duration of present residence. In addition, the head of the household has to furnish details of the residence including its type, tenure, accommodation and facilities. In recent years, it has been the practice to ask for additional information from a sample of the population. All the information relating to individuals is confidential, even within government departments.

Before census day, officials deliver the appropriate census form to each household and institution in the country. They are collected by the same official after census day, who is available to help householders with any problems they encounter. The data on the forms are analysed centrally by computer. In the past, tabulations of census data have been published as books, some of the more detailed information only after a delay of several years because of the time required for analysis and printing. The 1981 census was published both as books and as computer-readable magnetic tape. Despite some problems arising from concealment or misreporting of census information, and slight under-recording because some people are not at a formal address on census night, modern censuses are regarded as being generally very accurate.

ESTIMATES OF POPULATION BETWEEN CENSUSES

The size and demographic characteristics of the population in non-census years is estimated by deducting deaths and emigrants from numbers recorded in the census, and adding births and immigrants. At the same time, the age distribution of the people remaining is adjusted. These are known as *intercensal estimates*. Unfortunately errors occur which are compounded by the passage of time. The principle sources of error in the intercensal estimates arise through inadequate recording of immigration and emigration both in numbers and in respect of age and sex. Furthermore, there is no system for ascertaining the amount of internal migration (changes of residence within the country). Thus, the greater the time that has elapsed since a census, the less the precision of the estimate, especially estimates relating to small areas within the country. After a census, the figures for years since the last census are recalculated, taking account of the information provided by the new census. These are called *postcensal estimates*.

POPULATION PROJECTIONS

For planning purposes, it is often essential to have some idea of the likely size and composition of the population in years to come. The essential difference between population estimates and population projections is that an estimate is based on knowledge of the births, deaths and migration that have happened, and a projection is based upon what is thought likely to happen. Therefore, assumptions have to be made about trends in mortality, birth rates and migration. These are arrived at by extrapolation of past trends. Unforeseen changes in, for example, fertility can invalidate the projections.

VITAL EVENTS

General

Since the early nineteenth century, there has been a statutory requirement for all births, deaths and marriages in the UK to be registered. Before the Births, Marriages and Deaths Act (1839) most of the records that existed were kept by the ecclesiastical authorities. Since the vast majority of people at that time were baptized in infancy, the numbers of baptisms recorded in the parish registers can be used as proxy indicators of the numbers of live births. There was no information on stillbirths. As most marriages were in church, marriage rates also can be computed from the parish records. Likewise, most of the population received Christian burials and therefore the fact of death was usually recorded. However, the presumed cause of death was of little interest to the ecclesiastical authorities and was not routinely noted. In the seventeenth century, 'Bills of Mortality' were published for some large towns and cities. The best known are those compiled by John Graunt (Fig. 8.1). The cause of death was arrived at by paying lay 'searchers', normally women parishioners, to inspect the bodies and form an opinion. Whereas many of the common causes of death left stigmata that were plain for all to see, for example plague and smallpox, other diseases gave rise to less definite changes and there was doubtless considerable guesswork on the part of the searchers.

When the secular authorities made the registration of vital events mandatory, a government department called the Registrar General's Office was established to supervise the processing and collation of records, and to report to Parliament and other government depart- ments. Dr William Farr was the first medical statistician at the office. His meticulous and imaginative analyses of the data set the standards for the present sophisticated system for the registration, analysis and publication of vital events. Now the task of collating, analysing and publishing information relating to vital events is the responsibility of the OPCS.

Births

All births must be registered by one of the parents (or someone on their behalf) with the local Registrar of Births, Marriages and Deaths within 6 weeks of the event. Certain of the information required at this time is entered in the register and is available for public scrutiny. The following information is available for public scrutiny.

BIRTH REGISTRATION

- Child's name, sex, date and place of birth
- Mother's name, place of birth and usual residence
- Father's name (if known), place of birth and occupation

Not all of these data are entered on the birth certificate. Additional confidential information is collected for statistical purposes. This includes

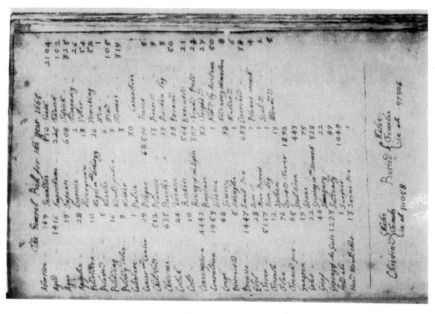

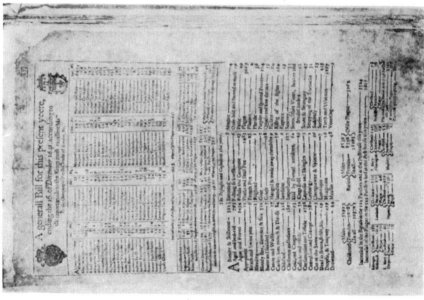

Fig. 8.1 The General Bills of Mortality for London, 1641 and 1665.

mother's date of birth and father's date of birth (if his name appears on the register). For legitimate births, the following additional information is required: date of parents' marriage, number of previous marriages of the mother and number of children born in the present marriage, distinguishing those born dead from those born alive.

If the child is stillborn, a certificate of cause of stillbirth has to be presented to the registrar. This certificate is similar to a death certificate and is issued either by a registered medical practitioner or by a state-certified midwife involved with the birth.

Tabulations and analyses of birth data are published annually by OPCS. They are used to study patterns of fertility and to assist in making population estimates and projections.

Deaths

The present regulations governing registration of deaths were set out in the Births and Deaths Registration Act (1968). The Act requires that: '. . . in the case of the death of any person who has been attended during his last illness by a registered medical practitioner, that practitioner shall sign a certificate . . . stating to the best of his knowledge and belief the cause of death and shall forthwith deliver that certificate to the Registrar.'

The certificate that the doctor is required to complete and sign (Fig. 8.2) is one of cause (or causes) of death, not of fact, since the doctor is not obliged to inspect the body after death. After giving the deceased's name, age, date and place of death and details of how far the death was investigated, the doctor is required to state the 'immediate cause' of death. There is then space provided for him or her to record the 'antecedent causes' (giving the 'underlying cause' last) and any other significant conditions that may have contributed to the death. As far as possible, the doctor should use generally accepted terminology, such as that set out in the ICD. The Registrar requires him or her to avoid the use of indefinite and ambiguous terms such as 'heart failure' or 'old age'. The completion of the certificate is quite straightforward in the case of an individual who has died as a result of a well-defined disease that has been extensively investigated in life, for example death by bronchopneumonia due to carcinomatosis due to carcinoma of the bronchus, with chronic bronchitis as a significant condition that contributed to death. However, in many circumstances the death certificate cannot be completed with such precision, for example in the case of an old person who has previously had a stroke, has diabetes, has chronic cardiac failure, is known to have bronchitis, has been bedridden for months and who is found dead in bed one morning. In such cases, the certified cause of death is an arbitrary opinion rather than a statement of fact. Generally, the precision of death certification tends to diminish with increasing age of the deceased.

An informant, who is usually a close relative of the deceased, a person present at death, the person in charge of the institution in which the person died or the person responsible for the disposal of the body, must register the death with the Registrar as soon after death as possible. When doing so, he or she must give the following information.

• Date and place of death
• Full name and sex of deceased
• Maiden name of married woman
• Date and place of birth of deceased
• Occupation and usual address of deceased

The data above are recorded in the register. If the Registrar is satisfied that the particulars are in order and that there is no need to report the death to the Coroner, he or she will issue a death certificate and authority for burial.

Death registration data are collated and analysed by the OPCS. The causes of death that are analysed are normally those given as the 'underlying cause' rather than the immediate cause because the former is more informative and more useful for the study of disease in the community. In the first example given above, the death would be classified as due to carcinoma of the bronchus for purposes of statistical analysis. The tables published by OPCS must be interpreted with this rule in mind. They do not necessarily provide a complete picture of mortality attributable in whole or part to specific causes.

In certain circumstances, a normal death certificate cannot be issued. These are when there was no medical attendant during the last illness of the deceased, when it is suspected that the death resulted from unnatural causes, or when the death occurred before full recovery from a surgical operation or the administration of an anaesthetic. In such circumstances, the death must be reported to the Coroner either by the attending doctor, or the police or the Registrar. A Coroner is a member of the judiciary and is bound by legal processes. He or she has to be legally qualified but not necessarily medically qualified, though some have both qualifications. The Coroner investigates the death by enquiry, either directly or through his or her officers. The Coroner may order a post-

Side 1

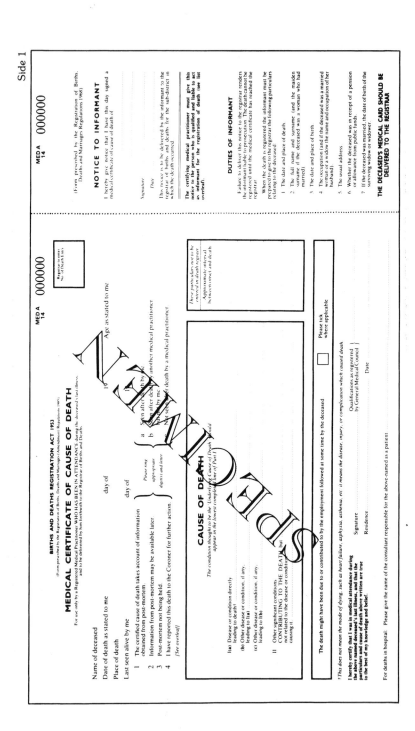

MEDA 14   000000

MEDICAL CERTIFICATE OF CAUSE OF DEATH

BIRTHS AND DEATHS REGISTRATION ACT 1953

(Form prescribed by the Registration of Births, Deaths and Marriages (Amendment) Regulations 1985)

For use only by a Registered Medical Practitioner WHO HAS BEEN IN ATTENDANCE during the deceased's last illness, and to be delivered by him forthwith to the Registrar of Births and Deaths.

Name of deceased

Date of death as stated to me   day of   19

Place of death

Last seen alive by me   day of

Age as stated to me

1 The certified cause of death takes account of information obtained from post-mortem.
2 Information from post-mortem may be available later
3 Post-mortem not being held
4 I have reported this death to the Coroner for further action.
   [See overleaf]

Please ring   a   Seen after death by me
appropriate   b   Seen after death by another medical practitioner
digit(s) and letter   Not seen after death by a medical practitioner

CAUSE OF DEATH

The condition thought to be the Underlying Cause of Death should appear in the lowest completed line of Part I

I(a) Disease or condition directly leading to death†

(b) Other disease or condition, if any, leading to I(a)

(c) Other disease or condition, if any, leading to I(b)

II Other significant conditions CONTRIBUTING TO THE DEATH but not related to the disease or condition causing it

These particulars not to be entered in death register

Approximate interval between onset of and death

The death might have been due to or contributed to by the employment followed at some time by the deceased

Please tick where applicable

† *This does not mean the mode of dying, such as heart failure, asphyxia, asthenia, etc. It means the disease, injury, or complication which caused death*

Qualifications as registered by General Medical Council

I hereby certify that I was in medical attendance during the above named deceased's last illness, and that the particulars and cause of death above written are true to the best of my knowledge and belief.

Signature

Residence   Date

For deaths in hospital. Please give the name of the consultant responsible for the above-named as a patient

MEDA 14   000000

Register to enter No. of Death here.

(Form prescribed by the Registration of Births, Deaths and Marriages Regulations 1968)

NOTICE TO INFORMANT

I hereby give notice that I have this day signed a medical certificate of cause of death of

Signature

Date

This notice is to be delivered by the informant to the registrar of births and deaths, for the sub-district in which the death occurred.

The certifying medical practitioner must give this notice to the person who is qualified and liable to act as informant for the registration of death (see list overleaf).

DUTIES OF INFORMANT

Failure to deliver this notice to the registrar renders the informant liable to prosecution. The death cannot be registered until the medical certificate has reached the registrar.

When the death is registered the informant must be prepared to give to the registrar the following particulars relating to the deceased

1 The date and place of death
2 The full name and surname (and the maiden surname if the deceased was a woman who had married)
3 The date and place of birth
4 The occupation (and if the deceased was a married woman or a widow the name and occupation of her husband)
5 The usual address
6 Whether the deceased was in receipt of a pension or allowance from public funds.
7 If the deceased was married, the date of birth of the surviving widow or widower

THE DECEASED'S MEDICAL CARD SHOULD BE DELIVERED TO THE REGISTRAR

Side 2

Complete where applicable

A

I have reported this death to the Coroner for further action.

Initials of certifying medical practitioner.

The Coroner needs to consider all cases where:

The death might have been due to or contributed to by a violent or unnatural cause (including an accident);

or the cause of death cannot be identified;

or the death might have been due to or contributed to by drugs, medicine, abortion or poison.

B

I may be in a position later to give, on application by the Registrar General, additional information as to the cause of death for the purpose of more precise statistical classification.

Initials of certifying medical practitioner.

or there is reason to believe that the death occurred during an operation or under or prior to complete recovery from an anaesthetic or arising subsequently out of an incident during an operation or an anaesthetic;

or the death might have been due to or contributed to by the employment followed at some time by the deceased

LIST OF SOME OF THE CATEGORIES OF DEATH WHICH MAY BE OF INDUSTRIAL ORIGIN

MALIGNANT DISEASES	Causes include	INFECTIOUS DISEASES	Cases include
(a) Skin	– radiation and sunlight – pitch or tar – mineral oils	(a) Anthrax	imported bone, bonemeal, hide or fur
(b) Nasal	– wood or leather work – nickel	(b) Brucellosis	farming or veterinary
(c) Lung	– asbestos – nickel – radiation	(c) Tuberculosis	contact at work
		(d) Leptospirosis	farming, sewer or undergroundworkers
(d) Pleura	– asbestos	(e) Tetanus	farming or gardening
(e) Urinary Tract	– benzidine – dyestuff – chemicals in rubbers	(f) Rabies	animal handling
(f) Liver	– PVC manufacture	(g) Viral hepatitis	contact at work
(g) Bone	– radiation	BRONCHIAL ASTHMA AND PNEUMONITIS	
(h) Lymphatics and haematopoietic	– radiation – benzene	(a) Occupational asthma	sensitising agent at work
POISONING		(b) Allergic Alveolitis	farming
(a) Metals	e.g. arsenics, cadmium, lead	PNEUMOCONIOSIS	
(b) Chemicals	e.g. chlorine, benzene		mining and quarrying potteries
(c) Solvents	e.g. trichlorethylene		asbestos

NOTE:—The Practitioner, on signing the certificate, should complete, sign and date the Notice to the Informant, which should be detached and handed to the Informant. The Practitioner should then, without delay, deliver the certificate itself to the Registrar of Births and Deaths for the sub-district in which the death occurred. Envelopes for enclosing the certificates are supplied by the Registrar.

PERSONS QUALIFIED AND LIABLE TO ACT AS INFORMANTS

The following persons are designated by the Births and Deaths Registration Act 1953 as qualified to give information concerning a death:—

DEATHS IN HOUSES AND PUBLIC INSTITUTIONS

(1) A relative of the deceased, present at the death.

(2) A relative of the deceased, in attendance during the last illness.

(3) A relative of the deceased, residing or being in the sub-district where the death occurred.

(4) A person present at the death.

(5) The occupier* if he knew of the happening of the death.

(6) Any inmate if he knew of the happening of the death.

(7) The person causing the disposal of the body.

DEATHS NOT IN HOUSES OR DEAD BODIES FOUND

(1) Any relative of the deceased having knowledge of any of the particulars required to be registered.

(2) Any person present at the death.

(3) Any person who found the body.

(4) Any person in charge of the body.

(5) The person causing the disposal of the body.

*"Occupier" in relation to a public institution includes the governor, keeper, master, matron, superintendent, or other chief resident officer.

Fig. 8.2 Death certificate (England and Wales). (Reproduced with permission of the OPCS (Crown copyright).)

mortem examination and may hold an inquest, with or without a jury. Having established the cause of death to his or her satisfaction, the Coroner will then sign a death certificate. If the Coroner has reason to believe that death was caused by the unlawful action of another person, he or she is bound to forward the papers to the Director of Public Prosecutions. It should be noted that in these circumstances it is the Coroner's job to establish the cause of death, not who caused it.

If those responsible for the disposal of the body wish the deceased to be cremated, an additional certificate is required. The person wishing to have the body cremated has to complete part of a form. The practitioner who attended the deceased during the last illness completes another part. This part has certain similarities to a certificate of cause of death but the doctor must have inspected the body after death. The third part is completed by another medical practitioner who is not professionally associated with the attending practitioner nor related to him or her or to the deceased. He or she must have been on the Medical Register for at least 5 years. This second doctor must inspect the body and form the view that the cause of death is as stated by the other practitioner. The final part is completed by the medical referee of crematoria for the local government authority involved. He or she has to affirm that the particulars on the other parts of the form are reasonable and have been completed by properly qualified doctors.

Stillbirths and infant deaths

Epidemiologists are particularly interested in the rate of stillbirths and infant deaths because they are a sensitive indicator of the general health of the population and also reflect the quality of child health services. Comparison of death rates between countries and the associated trends over time are of special interest. So that such comparisons can be made, agreed definitions and terminology have been promulgated by the WHO. (See box, opposite.)

The Still-birth (Definition) Act (1992) reduced from 28 weeks to 24 weeks the minimal gestational age by which a stillbirth is defined. This has increased the stillbirth and perinatal death rates. The infant death rate in the UK has fallen from around 150 per 1000 live births in 1900 to around 7 per 1000 in 1991. The current very low rate limits the possibility of further improvements. The commonest causes of neonatal death include

WHO DEFINITIONS

- Neonatal death   A live-born infant that dies within 28 days
- Early neonatal death   A live-born infant that dies within 7 days
- Late neonatal death   A live-born infant that dies after 7 days but within 28 days
- Stillbirth   A fetus that dies before birth but after a presumed 24 weeks of gestation
- Perinatal death   A combination of stillbirths and early neonatal deaths
- Postneonatal death   Deaths from 1 month to 1 year of age
- Infant deaths   Deaths under 1 year of age

congenital abnormalities and prematurity. Many of these deaths would seem to be unavoidable, although congenital rubella is one example which it is hoped can be completely eliminated. Around 40% of postneonatal deaths are due to cot death (sometimes called 'sudden infant death syndrome'). Associations have been shown with maternal smoking, prone sleeping position, bottle feeding and season of the year. A campaign to encourage mothers to place their baby on their side or back rather than prone has led to reduction in the number of cot deaths. The effectiveness of stopping smoking and encouraging breast feeding in reducing the number of deaths from cot death has yet to be shown. A small but increasing proportion of deaths in the postneonatal period are due to congenital abnormalities and conditions originating in the perinatal period suggesting that some infants that previously died soon after birth are now living until the postneonatal period.

Abortions

An abortion is the expulsion of the product of conception before it has reached an age when it could be expected to have an independent life and shows no signs of life at birth. The lower limit of fetal viability is defined as 24 weeks gestation. Since the Abortion Act (1967) came into force, it has been permissible for a pregnancy to be terminated provided it has not progressed beyond 28 weeks gestation, if two doctors believe that the continuation of the pregnancy would be injurious to the physical or mental health of the woman or that there is a risk that the child may be born with a disability that would prevent it from leading a normal life. Under 1990 legislation, abortion is normally permissible only up to 24 weeks gestation. When a termination of pregnancy is carried out under the provision of the Act (it is illegal to terminate a pregnancy other than for reasons set out in the Act) the doctors involved have a statutory obligation to notify the DoH. The form of notification asks for the name, date of birth and marital status of the woman, her normal place of residence, and the number of previous pregnancies, distinguishing those that proceeded to term from those that were terminated. The presumed duration of the pregnancy, the statutory grounds for the operation and the place where it was carried out are also required. The forms are sent in confidence to the DoH where they are checked to ensure that the law is not being abused. They are collated and analysed by the OPCS, which publishes annual tabulations setting out the number of abortions by different criteria.

MORBIDITY

General

Morbidity statistics are concerned with the amount and types of illness that occur in the community. The sources of available data vary from place to place and from time to time. They include, for example, attendances for primary care, hospital out-patients and admissions, as well as statutory sources and special registers for particular conditions. Most routinely collected morbidity data suffer from serious shortcomings partly because of the ephemeral nature and imprecise diagnosis of many illnesses and partly because of inadequacies in the information systems. Consequently, although they should give a more complete picture of the incidence of disease in communities than mortality data, they do so with varying reliability and must be interpreted with caution.

One of the principal problems centres around the definition of illness itself. For some people, a common cold or backache may represent an 'illness' and justify them seeking medical help or being away from work. These people's illnesses may be recorded in one of the many routine data systems. For other people, symptoms that the medical profession would regard as indicative or diagnostic of major disease may be regarded as having no serious significance, an inconvenience to be tolerated until normal recovery takes place. Such illnesses will not feature in any morbidity statistics because those affected do not seek medical aid nor allow the symptoms to alter their lifestyle.

Another problem is that diagnostic precision varies between doctors according to their perception of the disease that they are treating. For example, influenza and upper respiratory viral infections in most people are minor, self-limiting conditions for which there is no specific treatment. Diagnostic precision is unnecessary and it is a waste of time to attempt to discriminate between the many causes by complicated and expensive viral studies and other examinations. In such circumstances the data that are generated may not have sufficient precision for epidemiological studies.

In many cases, the stage at which disease is treated depends on a complex series of factors other than the patient's perception of the problem. These include the availability of health service treatments, for example waiting lists, out-patient appointment availability and the acceptability of the treatments that the patient believes will be offered. This will affect the morbidity recorded at hospitals and employment sickness absence figures.

Finally, there is a quite separate problem in the way morbidity statistics are calculated and presented. The calculation of mortality rates is relatively straightforward because each individual can only die once. Thus, if there are 10 deaths in a population of 162, the death rate is 61.7 per 1000. If, however, 10 episodes of an illness occur amongst 162 people during a year it does not mean that 61.7 per 1000 population were ill—one individual may have had more than one episode of illness; indeed, all the episodes may have occurred in the same individual. Many morbidity statistics are collected in such a way that it is impossible to distinguish episodes of illness from sick individuals. When presenting or making use of rates it is important to be clear how the rate was derived. Morbidity statistics routinely available in England and Wales include the following.

MORBIDITY STATISTICS

- Statutory notifications of infectious diseases
- Notification of episodes of STDs
- Notification of 'prescribed' and other industrial disease and accidents
- Notification of congenital malformations
- Cancer registration
- Laboratory reports on infections

Infectious diseases

When a doctor suspects that a patient is suffering from a notifiable infectious disease or from food poisoning (Table 8.1) the law requires him or her to send a certificate to the Proper Officer designated by the local authority. The officer responsible for infectious disease control is usually the local CCDC employed by the DHA. When it is a disease that is likely to require urgent control measures to be taken, the doctor will normally notify the CCDC by telephone and provide the formal certificate later. Similar action will usually be taken in the case of non-notifiable infectious diseases (or outbreaks due to other causes, for example chemical poisoning) which may require immediate investigation although this is usually undertaken by the environmental health officer employed by the local authority.

The importance of complete and prompt notification is not universally appreciated and therefore many infectious diseases are under-reported. Notification is important for a variety of purposes. In the case of some infections, such as food- and water-borne disease (food poisoning, typhoid, etc.), bacterial meningitis (particularly meningococcal infection), infectious hepatitis, diphtheria and tuberculosis, immediate action may be required to limit the spread of infection and to safeguard public health. Notifications are also of value in studying the aetiological factors influencing the incidence of disease in the community and in monitor-

NOTIFIABLE DISEASES

Under the Public Health (Control of Disease) Act (1984)

Cholera	Smallpox
Plague	Typhus
Relapsing fever	

Under the Public Health (Infectious Diseases) Regulations (1988)

Acute encephalitis	Ophthalmia neonatorum
Acute poliomyelitis	Paratyphoid fever
Anthrax	Rabies
Diphtheria	Rubella
Dysentery (amoebic or bacillary)	Scarlet fever
Leprosy	Tetanus
Leptospirosis	Tuberculosis
Malaria	Typhoid fever
Measles	Viral haemorrhagic fever
Meningitis	Viral hepatitis
Meningococcal septicaemia	Whooping cough
(without meningitis)	Yellow fever
Mumps	

Table 8.1 Statutorily notifiable infectious diseases.

ing the effectiveness of vaccination and immunization and other programmes.

Notifications of episodes of STDs

Genito-urinary medicine clinics of the NHS are required to make regular returns to the Department of Health for England (or its equivalent in other countries of the UK) of the numbers of new attendances with STDs. The following are defined as STDs for this purpose.

SEXUALLY TRANSMITTED DISEASES

Syphilis	Herpes simplex
Gonorrhoea	Condylomata acuminata
Non-specific genital infection	Molluscum contagiosum
Trichomoniasis	Chancroid
Candidiasis	Lymphogranuloma venereum
Scabies	Granuloma inguinale
Pediculosis pubis	Other attendances requiring treatment

For two of the above diseases, syphilis and gonorrhoea, the age of the patient and whether the disease was contracted outside the country has to be stated. In no case are data given that could identify an individual.

Although this system provides a useful picture of the overall trends in STD it has to be appreciated that not all cases treated are seen in NHS clinics. The nature of the information that is collected means that it is of limited value for all but the most basic of epidemiological studies. In particular, it is not possible to distinguish episodes from numbers of people involved. Notifications of HIV infection or AIDS are not included in clinic reports. Details of cases of AIDS are reported separately in confidence to the Director of the CDSC of the PHLS, which also collates reports from laboratories on HIV antibody-positive cases.

Industrial diseases and accidents

In order to improve personal safety at places of work, the HSE was established as a statutory body in 1974. Doctors are required to inform the Proper Officer, who in this instance may be the CEHO of the local authority or the CCDC, of the occurrence of any of the notifiable diseases they list. Doctors must also report poisoning by the following substances.

INDUSTRIAL POISON REPORTING

Aniline	Compressed air
Arsenic	Chrome
Benzene (chronic)	Lead
Beryllium	Manganese mercury
Cadmium	Phosphorous
Carbon bisulphide	

Also cases of epitheliomatosis, toxic anaemia and toxic jaundice

The HSE publishes the number of reported cases annually. Although the system is of great value in controlling these diseases, it undoubtedly gives an underestimate of the true incidence of these conditions. Many of the diseases occur in factories and work places in which there is no medical officer and, even if detected by another doctor, they are not always reported.

Employers also have an obligation to notify the HSE of accidents (both fatal and non-fatal) which occur in their factories or work place. These are published in the annual report.

A third source of data relating to industrial diseases is notifications of 'prescribed' occupational diseases, for example pneumoconiosis in coal miners, tuberculosis in medical laboratory workers and mesothelioma in asbestos workers. Workers who have these diseases are entitled to compensation under current regulations. Thus, notification is probably more complete than for many other diseases since there is a potential advantage in doing so to the individual with the disease. There are currently about 50 'prescribed' occupational diseases.

Congenital malformations

A national scheme for the notification of congenital malformations was instituted in England and Wales in 1961 after an episode in which thalidomide was responsible for a major outbreak of limb deformities in the children of mothers who had taken the drug during early pregnancy. There is no statutory requirement on doctors or midwives to notify cases. One of the problems with these data is the definition of malformations. There is little difficulty in detecting a major malformation but some minor abnormalities may not be noticed, or if noticed are not deemed to be of sufficient importance to justify notification.

Cancer registration

Malignant disease has long been a major cause of morbidity and mortality in the UK and in most other countries. In order to study these diseases, it is essential to know the numbers of people affected by different forms of cancer and their survival rates. The system of cancer registration was set up specifically to facilitate research in this field. Each region of the NHS maintains a cancer register to which new cases are notified by hospitals and others. The OPCS also notifies each Regional Cancer Registry of all people who die from malignant disease in their region. Data from all regions are analysed further by the OPCS. Periodic official reports are published giving detailed tabulations of incidence, survival and mortality rates for various malignant diseases at different stages.

Laboratory reports

The CDSC of the PHLS receives weekly reports from microbiology laboratories in England and Wales on cases of laboratory-diagnosed infections. The amount of clinical and epidemiological data reported varies depending on the infection. Although the data are incomplete and lack denominators which prevents their use to calculate incidence rates, they provide a useful means of monitoring trends and detecting out-breaks. The CDSC also collects data related to infectious disease from other sources, for example reports of outbreak investigations and immunization statistics. These reports are collated and published in the *Weekly Communicable Disease Report*.

HEALTH INFORMATION SYSTEMS

Information systems are used to assemble facts and figures from a variety of sources for analysis. Their main purposes are to provide accurate knowledge of the incidence and prevalence of disease in a community which will assist in the organization and monitoring of its health services and in disease-surveillance activities. Ideally, every health event and every kind of health resource would be recorded in a systematic and instantly available form. In practice, this is neither possible nor desirable as it would require an enormously complex and expensive system which would be too slow and cumbersome to be of value. Most health information systems have been developed to meet particular needs. Nevertheless, the data are often inaccurate and the system does not always allow users' questions to be answered with ease. These shortcomings tend to bring systems into disrepute and the enthusiasm for collecting data (as well as making use of it) wanes.

Some of the commonly encountered problems of information systems are as follows.

INFORMATION SYSTEM PROBLEMS

- Lack of motivation among recorders
- Design of data-capture procedure
- Inflexibility in the system
- Irrelevance of analyses

Lack of motivation among recorders. Often a low priority is accorded to the task of record keeping. This leads to delays in completion and poor quality of records, for example inaccurate information, items missing or no record at all. For these reasons all arrangements for 'data capture', as it is called, should be simple to operate and create the minimum amount of work.

Design of data-capture procedure. The type of record needed for an information system is not always compatible with that required for clinical purposes. It is often possible, however, to use records made for other purposes if they are carefully designed, i.e. in standard format with provision for coding, etc. This requires a degree of collaboration between different interests which it is often hard to achieve.

Inflexibility in the system. The need for simplicity in records means that the number of items recorded has to be restricted. Some flexibility can be gained by allowing room on the record for additional items of local interest beyond a set of basic data required of all recorders.

Irrelevance of analyses. Users may feel that standard analyses tell them nothing new or are unhelpful in solving their problems. This tends to sap enthusiasm for the system.

In the design of a routine information system, therefore, the following requirements should be met.

- The intended uses of the system should be specified so that the data recorded will be appropriate to their purpose and the collection of irrelevant data can be avoided.
- The recording procedures should be standardized and the data collected should be easy to obtain, accurate and as complete as possible in

order that reliable comparisons can be made over periods of time and between different places.

• Data should be collected from all relevant sources for collation and analysis at a central point.

• There should be well-organized provision for data storage, updating, processing and retrieval.

• The system should be capable of providing answers to enquiries within the field for which it is designed, with speed and accuracy.

CHAPTER 9

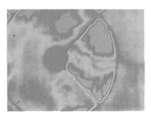

Indices of Health and Disease and Standardization of Rates

INTRODUCTION

The health of a community can be measured by the appropriate use of basic morbidity and mortality data, including those from sources described in the previous chapter. To be intelligible, however, the crude numbers need to be presented in a form that allows valid comparisons to be made between groups, between years and between different areas. There are certain conventions in the handling and presentation of data. There are four main types of variable as shown below.

- Qualitative.
- Ordinal.
- Continuous quantitative.
- Discrete quantititave.

TYPES OF VARIABLE

Qualitative variables

These are descriptive of a fixed attribute, for example sex, religion, occupation and nationality. Such data are sometimes classified for convenience by using numbers, e.g. 1 = male, 2 = female; or 1 = Church of England, 2 = Roman Catholic, 3 = Methodist, etc. These numbers have no meaning other than as labels.

Ordinal variables

These are used to rank the quality of characteristics in order of severity, importance, etc., for example pain might be classified as 0 = none, 1 = some pain, 2 = severe pain, 3 = very severe. The analysis of such variables requires different statistical techniques to quantitative variables.

Continuous quantitative variables

These measure attributes that can occur at any point on a scale, for example height, weight or blood pressure. The degree of precision to which a continuous variable is measured depends upon its intended use in a particular investigation and the discriminatory power of the measuring instrument.

Discrete quantitative variables

These measure attibutes that can occur only as whole numbers (integers), for example the number of children born to a woman or the number of deaths in a year.

GROUPING OF DATA

For convenience of handling and presentation, continuous variables may be grouped as if they were discrete. For example, the heights of people in a population may be grouped to the nearest centimetre so that all those whose height is over 122.5 cm and under 123.5 cm, all over 123.5 cm and under 124.5 cm, etc. can be assessed.

Discrete variables may also be grouped to produce larger numbers in each category. The class intervals between successive groups should usually be equal but it is often convenient to group all values at the extreme ends of a scale, which it must be remembered distorts the frequency distribution.

Situations in which groupings are natural should be distinguished from those where they are arbitrary, for example 'under 16 years' and '16 years and over' could be regarded as natural groupings in as much as people in the former category cannot be married and those in the latter can. For other variables, for example blood pressure, there is no such natural division. It is possible arbitrarily to define blood pressure in excess of 130 mmHg as high and below that level as not high, but this does not necessarily have any significance. Quantitative data rarely fall into natural categories.

RATES

It is rarely useful to state numbers of events observed and recorded alone. These can be interpreted only when they are related to a denominator, i.e. expressed as a rate, for example it is not helpful to say that the number of deaths from pneumoconiosis is greater in coal miners than in, say, farm workers without relating the figures to the numbers of people employed in the two occupations.

Two types of rate are frequently used: firstly events related to the population, or sub-group of it, in which they occur; and secondly special events related to total events.

Events related to the population

Examples
• Birth rates are usually given as x per 1000 total population per year.
• Age-specific rates relate the number of events in people in a specified age group to the total population in that age group, for example y deaths per 1000 men aged 45–64 years per year.
• Cause-specific rates relate cases of a specified disease to the population at risk, for example z cases of stroke per 1000 hypertensive patients per year.

Such rates must always have a specified time dimension.

Special events related to total events

Examples
• Stillbirths are usually expressed as x per 1000 total births.
• Operative mortality can be expressed as y deaths per 1000 operations.
• Case fatality rates relate the number of deaths from a particular illness to the total number of cases of that illness.

These types of rate are not time dimensioned because the time dimension is always the same for the numerator as it is for the denominator.

INCIDENCE AND PREVALENCE RATES

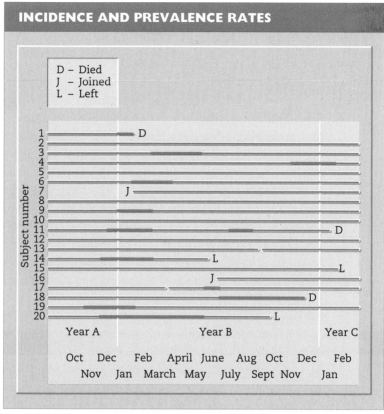

D – Died
J – Joined
L – Left

Fig. 9.1 Morbidity and mortality experienced in a hypothetical factory.

INCIDENCE AND PREVALENCE RATES

In order to demonstrate how incidence and prevalence rates are derived, the mortality and morbidity experience of the employees in a hypothetical factory is shown schematically in Fig. 9.1.

Incidence rates

The incidence of a disease or other events is the number of new cases that occur during a specified period in a defined population. Thus, from Fig. 9.1 in year B, the incidence of illness was 8. (The first illness in subject 11 and the illnesses in subjects 14, 19 and 20 started before the beginning of the period specified and are therefore discounted.) The incidence rate is eight per 18 people per year (by convention the mid-year population is used as the denominator). It should be noted that the incidence for a specific period is only valid for that period. Thus, in the 6 months January–June of year B, the incidence of disease was 5; it is clear that it cannot be multiplied to give an incidence of 10 during a 12-month period.

Prevalence rates

The prevalence of a disease is the number of cases in a defined population at a particular point in time (point prevalence) or during a specified period (period prevalence). Both are expressed as a rate (x per 1000 population). From Fig. 9.1, the point prevalence rate at the beginning of the year was four per 18 people and at the beginning of August it was two per 18 people (one had died and one had left since the beginning of the year and two had joined). The period prevalence for the year was 12 per 19 people (by convention the denominator is the mid-year population). The period prevalence approximates to the sum of the point prevalence at the beginning of the period and the incidence during the period.

ERROR IN HEALTH INFORMATION

The value of data ultimately depends on how accurately they reflect the true frequency of the disease (or other variable being measured) in the population concerned. This section sets out some of the common sources of error that may affect routine health information and the steps which can be taken to reduce their effects.

Errors affecting mortality and morbidity rates are of two kinds as shown below.

ERRORS AFFECTING MORTALITY AND MORBIDITY DATA

Those affecting the numerator, e.g.
- diagnostic inaccuracy
- incomplete identification of cases
- variability of the recording system

Those affecting the denominator, e.g.
- population migration
- changes in population structure
- changes in administrative boundaries

Numerator error

The number of recorded cases of a particular disease may be in error for many reasons including the following.

DIAGNOSTIC INACCURACY

This is affected by: the training, skills and interests of the attending physician; advances in medical knowledge of pathogenesis; variations in the criteria accepted in defining a diagnosis; differences in the availability and use of special investigations.

INCOMPLETE IDENTIFICATION OF CASES

The probability that patients will consult a doctor or be seen at or admitted to hospital, for example, is influenced by such factors as: past medical history; cultural and social background; occupation; economic constraints (e.g. paid sick leave); availability of medical care (which is related to numbers of doctors, distance from doctor's surgery, number of hospital beds and appointments systems). The effect of variations in illness behaviour is most marked in mild, non-fatal and self-limiting conditions.

THE RECORDING SYSTEM

The completeness and comparability of different sources of data may be affected by: the doctor's view of the value of records; the simplicity and efficiency of a records system; changes in the conventions for coding and classification of disease or rules for selecting priorities among multiple diagnoses.

Denominator error

The size of population at risk often cannot be defined accurately and various methods of estimation have to be used. Some reasons for this are:

• population migration between censuses may increase or decrease the size of population within an area;

• changes in population structure within different areas (e.g. age, race, occupational distribution), due to migration, changing fertility patterns, housing and industrial decay or development;

• changes in administrative boundaries for reasons that may or may not relate to health and the provision of health services.

Reduction of error

The effects of errors such as those above can be reduced as follows.

• By use of a standard diagnostic classification such as the ICD when recording mortality or modifications of this for morbidity.

• By combination of diagnostic categories between which transposition of cases may occur, e.g. cancer of the colon and large bowel obstruction.

• By use of standard recording and registration procedures.

• By use of denominator populations derived from similar sources and compiled by comparable procedures.

Errors in routine statistics can rarely be completely eliminated. Therefore, caution is needed in their interpretation, particularly between different localities and at different times (see also Chapter 4).

STANDARDIZATION OF RATES

Rates calculated by using the total number of events as the numerator and the total population as the denominator are called crude rates. Their value is limited, particularly when comparing two populations with different age structures, for example mortality rates in a new housing development with many young families and those in a coastal resort with a large retired population. In these circumstances, it is essential to adjust the data to take account of the differences; this is called age standardization. The two methods of standardization most frequently used are indirect standardization and direct standardization.

Indirect standardization

The conventional method of indirect standardization for age is to calculate the SMR. The SMR compares the mortality (either from a specific disease or for all causes) which occurred in a designated group with that of a standard population. It is the ratio (usually expressed as a percentage) of the number of deaths which occurred in the designated group to the number that would have been expected if the mortality rates in each age band of the designated group had been the same as those of the standard population.

Thus, the death rates for each age and sex group in the standard population (Mx) are multiplied by the number of people of that age and sex in the population being investigated (Px). This gives the 'expected' number of deaths in that particular age/sex group. The expected deaths for each age/sex group are then added to give the 'expected' number of deaths in the whole population being investigated. The observed number of deaths (D) is then divided by the expected deaths to give the SMR:

$$\text{SMR} = \frac{\text{observed deaths} \left(D \right)}{\text{expected deaths} \left[\Sigma \left(P_x \times M_x \right) \right]} \times 100$$

Example: members of the armed forces tend to be younger than the male population of the country as a whole. Therefore, the fact that they have a lower mortality rate is not illuminating. It is necessary to examine the mortality of this occupational group after taking account of the age factor. Their SMR for IHD is calculated in Table 9.1. This indicates that mortality from IHD amongst men in the armed forces after adjusting for age distribution is higher than the national experience by a factor of 1.73.

Another example of how standardization can be helpful is in comparing mortality in different years. The age structure of the population of England and Wales has been changing for many years and therefore crude death rates can give a misleading impression of changes in mortality. The SMR gives a clearer indication of the true picture (Table 9.2). This

IHD DEATHS IN MILITARY MEN

Age group (years)	Death rates from IHD in England and Wales (per 1000) (M_x)	Population of armed services (1000s) (P_x)	Expected deaths ($M_x \times P_x$)	Observed deaths
15–24	0	165.03	0	1
25–34	0.06	73.24	4.39	6
35–44	0.50	42.25	21.13	22
45–54	2.01	15.93	32.02	43
55–64	6.05	4.67	28.75	76
Total			85.79	148

$$\text{SMR} = \frac{\text{observed}}{\text{expected}} \times 100 = \frac{148 \times 100}{85.79} = 173$$

Note: SMRs for occupational sub-groups are usually confined to people aged 15–64 years because the working population is confined to this age group.

Table 9.1 Mortality from IHD in men serving in the armed forces.

INDIRECT STANDARDIZATION

Age group (years)	Death rate (per 1000) males in England and Wales, 1965 (M_x)	Male population in England and Wales (1000s), 1973 (P_x)	Expected deaths ($P_x \times M_x$)	Observed deaths
<1	21.8	355.3	7 746.0	
1–4	0.9	1 561.7	1 406.0	
5–14	0.5	4 037.3	2 019.0	
15–24	1.0	3 534.2	3 534.0	
25–34	1.1	3 337.5	3 671.0	
35–44	2.5	2 877.6	7 194.0	
45–54	7.4	3 033.6	22 449.0	
55–64	21.4	2 643.1	56 562.0	
65–74	53.0	1 855.9	98 363.0	
75+	118.4	639.7	75 740.0	
85+	242.4	112.8	27 343.0	
Total			306 026.0	296 546

$$\text{SMR} = \frac{\text{observed}}{\text{expected}} \times 100 = \frac{296\,546}{306\,026} \times 100 = 97$$

Table 9.2 Mortality in males in England and Wales in 1965 compared with 1973.

DIRECT STANDARDIZATION

Age group	Population, 1949 (a) (1000s)	Deaths, 1949 (b)	Death rate, 1949 (b/a)	Population, 1979 (c) (1000s)	Expected (c × b/a)
0–9	3 417	17 643	5.16	3 339	17 231.3
10–19	2 869	2 345	0.82	4 063	3 331.7
20–29	3 339	5 031	1.51	3 534	5 336.3
30–39	3 189	6 839	2.14	3 326	7 117.6
40–49	3 178	16 062	5.05	2 020	14 241.0
50–59	2 335	32 097	13.75	2 924	40 205.0
60–69	1 727	60 580	35.08	2 257	74 661.6
70–79	957	77 127	80.59	1 384	111 536.6
80+	228	42 218	185.17	355	65 735.4
Total	21 239	260 278		24 002	339 396.5

Table 9.3 Standardization of mortality in England and Wales in 1949 against the 1979 population. The age-standardized 1949 death rate (against the 1979 population) is 339 396.5/24 002 = 14.14 per 1000. This can be compared directly with the crude death rate for 1979 which was 12.41 per 1000.

indicates that mortality in males in England and Wales declined between 1965 and 1973.

Direct standardization

Direct standardization for age involves calculating the age-specific death rates in the study population and applying them to the same age groups in a 'standard' population. This can be real or hypothetical. In this way, the number of deaths that would have occurred in the standard population, had it experienced the same death rates as the study population, can be computed and compared with other groups. The method of direct standardization is shown in Table 9.3.

CHAPTER 10

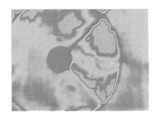

Medical Demography

INTRODUCTION

Despite the presence of many serious endemic diseases and the occurrence of major epidemics and wars, the populations of most European countries increased substantially during the past 300–400 years. There has been a reduction in the rate of increase in recent decades and today the populations of most European and North American countries are relatively stable. It seems likely that in the foreseeable future they will either remain stable or there might even be a modest decrease.

The growth of the European resident population since the seventeenth century underestimates both the extent to which the numbers of European people increased and the rate at which the increase took place. Throughout the past 400 years, people have emigrated in large numbers mainly to the Americas, Australasia and to parts of Africa. The migrations were prompted by economic hardship, social pressures and religious persecution as well as for trading reasons and fortune hunting. The majority of the present populations of North America and Australasia are descendants of these migrants. Their numbers now exceed those of the parent (European) populations.

Whether or not the European population would have increased in size to the extent that it has without migration and dispersal throughout the world can only be a matter of speculation. It is unlikely that it would have done, as the natural resources of Europe would have been insufficient to support so large a population. Furthermore, the technology to create a safe urban environment, with pure water, adequate sanitation and means for the bulk transport of food, did not exist until recently.

The populations of most other parts of the world began to increase much more recently and their rate of increase has reached that prevailing in Europe in the eighteenth and nineteenth centuries only during the past few decades. An important difference between the contemporary situation in many of the poorer developing countries of the world and Europe in previous centuries is that there are no longer large, sparsely populated continents rich in natural resources that can be colonized and in which people can thrive. Thus, population growth, which in previous generations was regarded as a national problem, is now a world problem. It is forecast that if the prevailing rates of growth are sustained, the world's population, now about 5700 million people, will double within the next 40 years. The earth's mineral and energy resources are finite and the rate at which they are being consumed is increasing, particularly by the industrialized countries. In many parts of the world, there is a hopeless inability to meet local needs, and resources are inadequate to enable them to import essential commodities. It is predicted that, unless there are reductions in both the rate of population growth and the rate at which natural resources are consumed, there will be a catastrophic failure to meet the basic needs of the majority of humankind within the next few generations.

Cataclysmic prophecies that humankind's future is threatened in this way are not new. They have been widely debated since the eighteenth century. Probably the best known writer associated with the problems of overpopulation is the Reverend Thomas Malthus, an eighteenth century English clergyman who attracted attention by his essay on 'The principles of population as it affects the future improvement of society'. The two principles from which he argued were: 'that food is necessary for the existence of man' and that 'the passion between the sexes is necessary and will remain nearly in its present state'. He argued that the power of the population to reproduce was greater than power of the earth to produce food. He concluded that there must be a 'strong and constantly operating check on population from the difficulty of subsistence'. This conclusion led him to recommend that there should be no extension of relief for the poor, as this would artificially reduce the difficulties of subsistence and lead to uncontrolled population growth. The time scale within which he predicted catastrophe was wrong, partly because he did not foresee emigration and colonization. His contention that difficulties in subsistence would act as a constant check on population growth has also been proved wrong by the experience in the countries of Latin America, the Indian subcontinent and elsewhere.

At about the same time as the ideas of Malthus were being debated in Europe, similar discussions were taking place in China. Hung Wang Chi noted in 1793 that 'during a long reign of peace the government cannot prevent people from multiplying themselves, yet its remedies are few'. One of the solutions that he suggested was to legalize and encourage female infanticide, a practice that continues in some parts of the world to this day. Discussions of the problems of population have continued throughout the world up to the present time but now more is known about the size of the world population, the dynamics of growth and the potential resources of the earth. The United Nations, through its various agencies, regards population growth as one of the major world problems that will affect the quality of life, health and survival of humankind.

The countries with high population growth are mainly developing countries where there are already regular famines, chronic poverty, frequent epidemics of crippling diseases and declining living standards. The situation will only be remedied if those countries with the highest growth rates in population achieve stability and the countries with the highest growth rates in consumption of resources reduce their demands.

The global problem of population growth is compounded by the fact that people are not evenly distributed on the habitable surface of the earth. Food shortages and disease are problems in some areas simply because of the local density of population rather than because the area as a whole has insufficient natural resources. It is important to recognize that health depends as much upon the systems for the distribution of food and water and the disposal of waste as it does upon the quantity of food produced or the availability of medical services.

POPULATIONS AND GROWTH RATES

The size of the world's population and its growth rate is arrived at by collating data from every country. The quality of the data varies considerably from country to country. Most of the richer industrialized countries undertake regular and detailed censuses similar to those undertaken in England and Wales (see p. 78). They also have sophisticated and comprehensive systems for the registration of births, deaths and marriages. From these sources it is possible to build up a complete picture of the way in which the size and structure of the population changes.

In the poorer countries of the world, national censuses are conducted infrequently and tend to be incomplete. The additional data that are required for demographic studies, the registration of vital events, are often defective. There are particular difficulties in the most deprived sections of these countries and amongst nomadic peoples or those living in sparsely populated regions of the world with poor communications. In these latter situations, much of the data are available only on an irregular sample basis. It is not surprising that most of the work on population growth has used European data, because only in recent times has it been possible to study many of the other countries of the world.

The trends in population growth in England and Wales are not dissimilar to those in most European countries and can be used to illustrate the size and speed at which changes occurred. It has proved possible to estimate the number of residents at various times between 1100 and the early nineteenth century from analysis of ecclesiastic l and gove nmental records. From the nineteenth century onwards form ' census f res are available. The trend has been for the population to inc exponentially (Fig. 10.1). The temporary decreases in population du to major national disasters such as epidemics of plague or war are not discernible within the scale used on the figure but at the time they had major impacts in some parts of the country. For example, Fig. 8.1 (p. 81) shows the 'General Bills of Mortality for London' for 1641 and 1665. In both years, the number of deaths greatly exceeded the number of births, in 1665 by

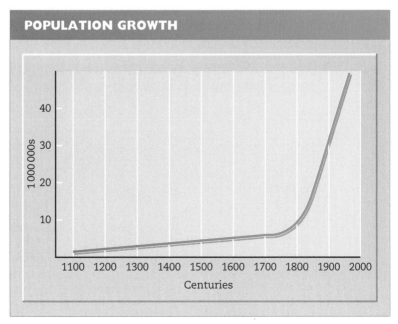

POPULATION GROWTH

Fig. 10.1 The growth of population in England and Wales.

a factor of 10. It should be remembered that Fig. 10.1 is solely concerned with the resident population and that during much of the period there was substantial migration. It should also be noted that the scale of the figure is such that the recent reduction in population growth rate is not apparent.

At the same time as the population increased, its age structure changed. Figure 10.2 compares the age distribution of the population in 1821 with that in 1991. In 1821, the proportion of children was much greater than at the present time and the proportion of people over the age of 50 was considerably less. The 1991 census showed that the proportion of the population between 20 and 29 years is greater than that in the age group 10–19 years. This is due in part to an increase in the number of births during the 1960s and in part to a reduction in birth rates in the 1970s.

The population can only increase if the number of births exceeds the number of deaths. The growth rate of human populations tends to be exponential because with each annual increase in births the proportion of the population potentially capable of reproduction increases. For this reason, the statement that there is an annual growth rate of x per 1000 population (x being the difference between the birth rate and the death rate) gives a misleading impression of the magnitude of change. The conventional way of expressing growth is the population doubling time. This is the theoretical period that it will take for a given population to double, based upon the most recently available data. Clearly, the doubling

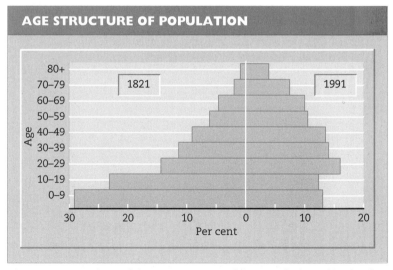

Fig. 10.2 Comparison of the age structure of the population of England and Wales in 1821 with that in 1991.

time will have to be revised when there is a change in either birth or death rate. The doubling time for the population of the UK, together with that for a number of other countries, is given in Table 10.1.

DEMOGRAPHIC TRANSITION

The model of demographic transition provides a useful framework within which to consider the factors which determine changes in the size and structure of human populations. The population is stable both in size and in age structure when the birth and death rates are equal and static, irrespective of whether they are both high or both low. This phase is

POPULATION DOUBLING TIMES

Country	Population (1000s)	Birth rate (per 1000)	Death rate (per 1000)	Population doubling time (years)	Life expectancy, males (years)	Life expectancy, females (years)	Fertility
Kenya	25 905	47.0	11.3	19.8	56.5	60.5	7.0
Cambodia	5 729	41.4	16.6	28.3	47.0	49.9	4.7
Mexico	81 141	29.0	5.8	30.2	62.1	66.0	4.2
Argentina	32 609	21.7	7.9	50.6	65.5	72.7	3.0
Singapore	2 705	17.8	5.0	54.5	68.7	74.0	2.0
New Zealand	3 380	17.8	7.8	69.6	71.9	78.0	2.2
India	844 324	29.9	20.3	72.5	55.4	55.7	4.0
Canada	25 309	15.3	7.3	87.0	73.0	79.8	1.8
USA	248 710	16.3	8.6	90.4	71.8	78.6	2.0
Ireland	3 523	14.9	8.9	115.9	71.0	76.7	2.2
Russian Fed.	143 585	14.6	10.7	178.1	64.2	74.5	2.0
Sweden	8 635	14.3	11.0	210.4	74.8	80.4	2.1
Japan	123 611	9.9	6.7	217.0	75.9	81.8	1.6
UK	57 367	13.8	11.3	277.6	72.4	78.0	1.8
Spain	39 025	10.2	8.5	408.1	73.2	79.1	3.7
Belgium	9 844	12.0	10.6	495.5	70.0	76.8	1.6
Denmark	5 148	12.4	11.9	1 386.6	71.8	77.7	1.6
Italy	57 052	9.8	9.3	1 386.6	73.2	79.7	1.3

World region	Population (millions)	Birth rate (per 1000)	Death rate (per 1000)	Population doubling time (years)
Africa	662	45.0	15.0	23.5
Latin America	457	29.0	7.0	31.9
Asia	3171	28.0	9.0	36.8
Oceania	27	19.0	8.0	63.4
Former USSR	291	18.0	11.0	99.4
North America	278	15.0	9.0	115.9
Europe	500	13.0	11.0	346.9
World	5385	27.0	10.0	41.1

Table 10.1 Population doubling times in various countries and regions of the world. (Source: WHO, 1991.)

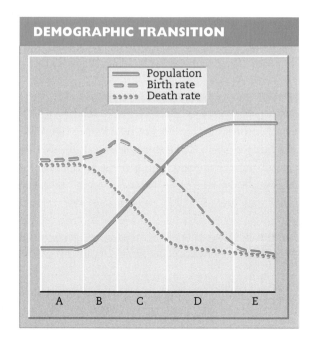

DEMOGRAPHIC TRANSITION

Population
Birth rate
Death rate

A   B   C   D   E

Fig. 10.3 Schematic representation of demographic transition.

represented in Fig. 10.3 as period A. Typically primitive rural societies and poorly developed urban societies tend to have high birth and high death rates. The highest mortality tends to be in infancy and childhood due to the combined effects of disease and poor nutrition.

Social progress and the introduction of industrial technology bring tangible and immediate benefits to the community. The most obvious are improvements in sanitation, in water supply and in the ability to distribute and store food. The immediate effect of these changes is that the chances of survival amongst the most vulnerable within the community, infants and children, are improved. Therefore the death rate begins to fall and the community enters phase B in Fig. 10.3. During this phase, the crude birth rate actually rises because the proportion of the population that is capable of reproduction increases and there is little change in the age-specific birth rates. This is because people's reproductive behaviour tends to be learned from their parents and it can take many years to adapt fully to new circumstances. In many societies, the desirability of large families, which is a biological necessity for survival in pretransitional communities, is formalized within the belief system of the group. For example, in many societies, the number of children a man has is perceived as a measure of his virility. The next phase (C in Fig. 10.3) is characterized by a decrease in the birth rate while the death rate continues to fall. Birth rates still exceed death rates and the exponential growth of the population, established in phase B, continues. Again this is because, despite a decrease in the average number of children born to each woman, there are more women in the reproductive age group than there were in the previous phase.

Eventually death rates stabilize (phase D) but birth rates continue to fall. The transition of the society is completed in phase E, when birth and death rates are static and equal. By this time, the size of the population is many times greater than it was in the pretransitional phase. The size of the new stable population is determined by the speed of the transition.

Data from England and Wales can be used to illustrate the demographic changes discussed above. The crude and the age-specific death rates for selected age groups relative to the 1841 rates in England and Wales are shown in Fig. 10.4. The crude death rate is now about half what it was in the early nineteenth century. The greatest changes in mortality have been amongst the young, exemplified by the 5–9 year olds in the figure, which are now less than 5% of the rates prevailing in the early nineteenth century. The smallest changes have been amongst the

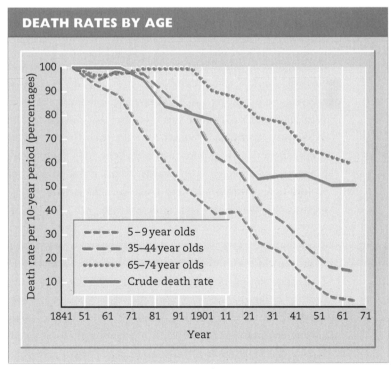

DEATH RATES BY AGE

Death rate per 10-year period (percentages)

- - - - 5–9 year olds
- - - 35–44 year olds
••••••• 65–74 year olds
——— Crude death rate

Year

Fig. 10.4 Age-specific death rates per 10-year period for England and Wales since 1841, as a percentage of the 1841–1850 age-specific rates.

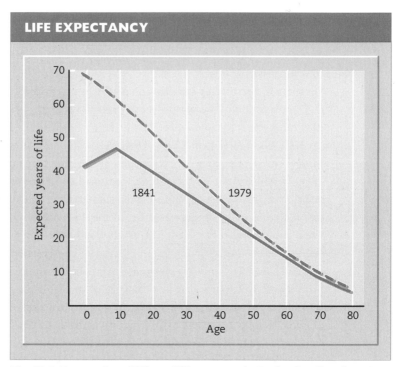

LIFE EXPECTANCY

Fig. 10.5 Expectation of life at different ages in England and Wales, 1841 and 1979.

elderly. This is reflected in the change in life expectancy, another way of summarizing mortality, at different ages (Fig. 10.5). It is arrived at by applying the prevailing age- and sex-specific mortality rates to the people who survive to a particular age. It is clear that the greatest changes in life expectancy have been amongst the very young. Increased survival in the prereproductive age groups means that the proportion of the population capable of reproduction increases. Thus, although each age group of women may maintain the same age-specific fertility rates as previous generations, the crude birth rates will rise.

REASONS FOR THE DECLINE IN MORTALITY

The reduction in mortality in England and Wales since the nineteenth century is almost entirely due to the elimination of the major endemic infectious diseases (Fig. 10.6). For most of these, mortality rates were highest amongst young people. It is apparent that the virtual disappearance of these diseases from the UK, and from most countries in the western world, owed more to improvements in the general quality of life and to improvements in public and personal hygiene than they did to any

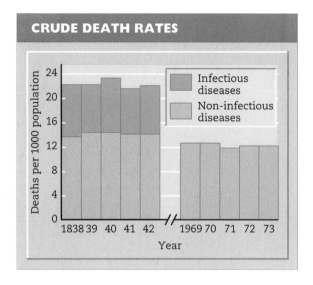

CRUDE DEATH RATES

Fig. 10.6 Crude annual death rates from infectious and non-infectious diseases in England and Wales, 1838–1842 and 1969–1973. (Death rates from infectious diseases during 1969–1973 were too low to show on this scale.)

specific medical measures. Specific medical treatments were not introduced until long after the mortality rates from these diseases had undergone the greater part of their fall. It is noteworthy that many of the lethal diseases of nineteenth-century Europe are now regarded as 'tropical diseases'. They are more properly called 'poverty diseases'. The principal diseases that accounted for the high mortality and which have now been controlled or eliminated in the western world were tuberculosis, the enteric fevers, cholera, smallpox, scarlet fever, measles, whooping cough and diphtheria.

During the 1840s, about 18% of all deaths in England and Wales were attributed to tuberculosis. It is possible that some of these may have been misdiagnosed carcinoma of the bronchus or some other disease of the respiratory system, but the numbers were so large that there can be little doubt that the downward trend in mortality rates shown in Fig. 3.1 (p. 21) was mainly a reflection of tuberculosis control. The decline in tuberculosis mortality preceded the identification of the organism or any specific treatment. The principal explanation for this remarkable trend, however, probably lies in improvements in diet and in consequent enhancement of the resistance of individuals. The practice of isolating cases, thereby reducing the spread of the disease, probably also had an effect.

The enteric and diarrhoeal diseases were endemic in the nineteenth century and were a particularly important cause of death amongst infants and children. Their impact began to decline in the 1870s (Fig. 10.7) and seemed to be the result of improvements in personal hygiene and in child-rearing practices. A more specific measure, the provision of a pure

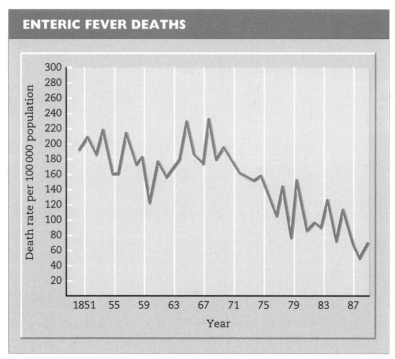

Fig. 10.7 Mortality rates from enteric fevers, England and Wales, 1851–89.

water supply, was responsible for the disappearance of cholera as an endemic disease in the UK (Fig. 10.8).

Because of the obvious physical signs of smallpox, the statistics on its mortality are likely to have been accurate. This disease was endemic in the nineteenth century (Fig. 10.9). Typically, there were superimposed regular epidemics every 6–7 years. The frequency of these epidemics was probably due to changes in population immunity. Contact with disease either resulted in death or life-long immunity, thereby reducing the size of the susceptible population. After an epidemic, most survivors would be immune and this decreased the risk to the remaining susceptibles. When the proportion of susceptibles in the population increased (by the birth of children), a further epidemic occurred. Not surprisingly, the majority of deaths occurred amongst children and infants. The elimination of this disease was due to a specific medical measure, the discovery of vaccination. However, it should be noted that although vaccination became compulsory in England in 1852, it was not widely practised for a further 20 years.

Other infectious diseases that ceased to be a major cause of mortality included scarlet fever, which was endemic and had regular superimposed

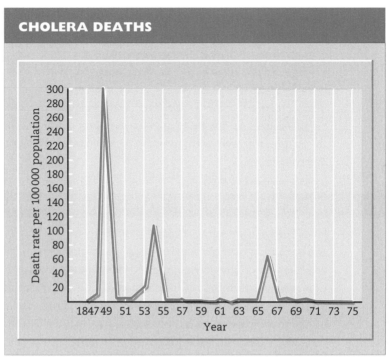

Fig. 10.8 Cholera mortality in England and Wales, 1847–77.

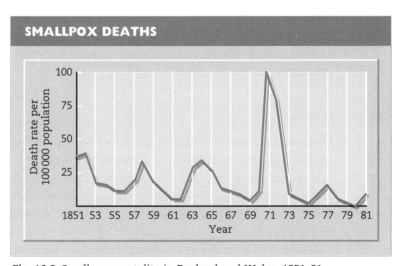

Fig. 10.9 Smallpox mortality in England and Wales, 1851–81.

epidemics. Its eventual elimination could have been due to the advent of more successful treatments for the complications of the disease or to changes in the virulence of the organism.

Many of the measures that have achieved the control of the infectious diseases are to a large extent by-products of improvements in the quality of life and, more recently, relatively simple medical measures. All should be applicable and are being applied in poorer countries of the world at the present time with consequent accelerating reductions in their mortality levels.

FACTORS AFFECTING FERTILITY IN COMMUNITIES

It has been shown that reductions in mortality have been achieved either as by-products of tangible and universally acceptable improvements in the environment or from certain specific medical measures, such as vaccination, which reduce the risk of contracting diseases. By contrast, reductions in the fertility of a population require the consent and cooperation of individuals together with changes in their personal attitudes to child bearing and child rearing. In pretransitional populations, it is necessary for women to bear large numbers of children in order that there will be sufficient survivors to maintain the size of the community and to provide a work force to sustain essential activities. Strong social customs and belief systems have grown up to support this need and, therefore, changes in fertility depend on changes in social customs and ethics. Next, it is necessary to promote and make available fertility control to individuals.

Social factors

By convention, child bearing and child rearing outside marriage have been discouraged in most societies. In contemporary western societies, this attitude has changed but in most of the world, powerful taboos remain and societies continue to censure the unmarried mother and her child. Thus, marriage practices have a potent effect on the reproductive behaviour of societies.

The legal minimum age of marriage is of less importance in most societies than the conventional age of marriage. It is, however, used as a means of reducing population growth in some countries, notably China, where it has recently been raised by 2 years. Although conception may still take place below the minimum age for marriage, the pregnancy is stigmatized as illegitimate. The conventional age of marriage tends to be several years greater than the legal minimum. In nineteenth-century Sweden, the conventional age of marriage was the middle to late twenties. This convention was imposed in rural communities by obliging a man to demonstrate his ability to support his wife before marriage could take place and by his living apart from women during the period he was becoming established. Although the age-specific legitimate fertility rates of Swedish women at this time were close to the maximum possible, the effective duration of the fertile period was reduced. In Ireland, there has always been a tendency for late marriage. In England and Wales there have been significant changes in the age of first marriage during the past 50 years (Table 10.2). The effect of the proportion of women who are married on age-specific birth rates is obvious from Table 10.3. The legitimate birth rate to women aged 20–24 was similar in 1939 and 1969 but the age-specific birth rates differ considerably because the proportion of women who were married changed.

Divorce, separation and widowhood have the reverse effect on birth rates to those of marriage. The same conventions that discourage never-

MARRIAGE RATES

| | Age in years | | |
	16–19	20–24	25–29
1938	28.1	171.6	132.2
1948	49.1	212.5	158.1
1958	75.2	260.8	162.5
1968	84.6	260.9	161.4
1978	58.8	177.9	134.8
1988	23.0	101.6	106.8

Table 10.2 First marriage rates per 1000 single women in England and Wales. (Source: Registrar General's Annual Statistical Reviews.)

BIRTH RATES

	Legitimate births per 1000 married women	Percentage of women who were married	Births per 1000 women (married and single)
1939	252	33	93
1969	251	58	157
1988	212	30	95

Table 10.3 Births to women aged 20–24 years in England and Wales. (Source: Registrar General's Annual Statistical Reviews.)

married women from having children, discourage divorced and widowed women from reproducing. In normal times, this has little impact on birth rates but, after World War I, when many women in Europe were widowed, there was a noticeable reduction in the number of births, although there had been little change in the size of the female population in the reproductive age group.

Sexual behaviour within marriage varies between societies. Although taboos exist regarding the permissibility of intercourse at certain times, for example during menstruation or religious feasts, this has little measurable effect on birth rates.

Contraception

Although the possibility of contraception and knowledge of techniques has existed for many years (it was known to and used by the ancient Egyptians), its use varies substantially from place to place depending on its acceptability, availability and efficiency.

Nowadays, in most societies, the most important social factor determining the patterns of reproduction is the acceptability of contraception. In general, the better educated (and those who are better off) are more likely to use contraception than the ill-educated and poor. Its use is also determined to some extent by religious beliefs. Members of the Roman Catholic Church are forbidden to use artificial methods of birth control. Nevertheless, the rule of the church is not universally adhered to and contraceptive practice varies amongst Roman Catholics. It has been shown that a large proportion of Roman Catholics in Europe and North America no longer adhere to their church's teaching.

The Roman Catholic Church is not the only religious group actively to discourage the practice of contraception. Within Christian cultures, the Hutterite and Amish communities take the Biblical dictum to go forth and multiply quite literally and amongst them it is not unusual for married women to produce a dozen or more children. Some non-Christian religious groups also eschew contraception on principle. Local ethics and morals may restrict the availability of the more efficient methods to certain groups. Thus, if sexual intercourse outside marriage is deemed wrong, contraception for the unmarried may be seen as a collusion with immorality. In the 1960s and 1970s, many clinics in England and some general practitioners would not advise unmarried women on contraception.

In societies where the role of women is seen mainly as child bearing and child rearing, women who limit their fertility may be rejected or may fear rejection. Similar problems affect the acceptability of contraception in groups where a man's success and strength is measured by the number of children he fathers. During transition between high and low mortality, fear of death of existing infants and children, resulting in the extinction of the family, leads to the production of more children. It is often difficult to convince parents in such societies that the survival of existing children is threatened by further enlargement of the family.

Even if the idea of birth control is acceptable to an individual, the method of contraception involved may be unacceptable. Many of the simpler methods require action by the male (e.g. the sheath or coitus interruptus), and they may detract from his satisfaction. The methods that require no action at the time of intercourse usually require intervention by trained professionals (e.g. the intrauterine device (IUD) or sterilization). The choice and use of methods of contraception is also affected by the couple's level of education. This is important in communities where birth control is new and where modern techniques are not common knowledge. Most developing countries have recognized this factor as important and are experimenting with teaching methods. The most effective methods are usually the most expensive. If family economics mean that people cannot afford the new technology then in practice the method is not available to them. The problem of cost is greatest in countries with the greatest problems.

The efficiency of a particular method of contraception is assessed by the number of conceptions per women-years of use. The assessment should be made in a group similar to that in which the method will be used. Table 10.4 shows estimates of relative efficiency of some of the current methods. These estimates were made in married women who were likely to have regular intercourse and to be motivated to use the method correctly. Some couples use contraceptive methods incorrectly. For example, there is some evidence that single women are erratic in their use of oral contraceptives which alters the apparent effectiveness of the method.

Table 10.4 The relative efficiency of different methods of contraception.

CONTRACEPTION EFFICIENCY

Contraceptive used	Pregnancies per 100 women-years of use
Oral contraceptives	0.15
Intra-uterine device	2.00
Diaphragm	2.40–5.00

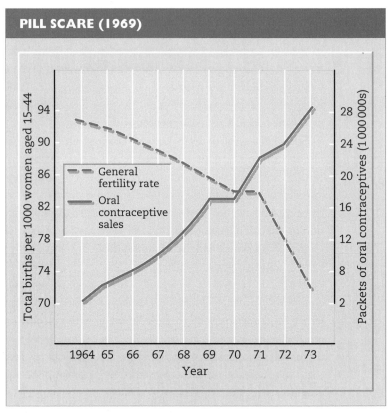

PILL SCARE (1969)

Fig. 10.10 General fertility rate and oral contraceptive sales, showing the effect of the 1969 'pill scare'.

In 1969, a great deal of publicity was given to the possible danger of producing venous thrombo-embolic disease by oral contraceptives and a large number of women precipitately stopped using them. They did not appear to use alternative methods and consequently the decline in birth rate in England and Wales was temporarily halted (Fig. 10.10).

SOME RECENT CHANGES IN THE PATTERNS OF FERTILITY IN ENGLAND AND WALES

For about 50 years until the 1980s, there was a tendency for women to marry earlier. Since then there has been a steady rise in the age of first marriage. The mean interval between first marriage and the birth of the first child fell until the early 1970s when it began to increase (Fig. 10.11).

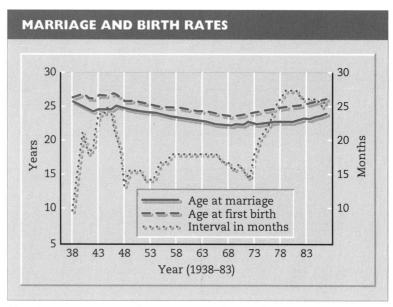

Fig. 10.11 Average age of women at marriage and average age at birth of first legitimate child in England and Wales.

The increase in the interval between first marriage and first pregnancy was associated with an increase in the use of efficient contraception, particularly oral contraception and the IUD. The mean interval between marriage and pregnancy is affected by the proportion of women who are pregnant when they marry. Figure 10.12 shows that in the 1960s about 40% of women who married under the age of 20 years and about 15% of women aged 20–29 years were pregnant when they married. The proportions fell in all age groups during the 1970s. The post-1970s changes were due to a combination of increased availability of abortion and of contraception to unmarried people. This hypothesis is consistent with the fall both in the illegitimate birth rate and in the number of marriages of pregnant women.

Figure 10.13 shows the cumulative age-specific fertility rates for cohorts of women born in different years. The 1920 and 1930 cohorts reached their peak birth rates at about the age of 26 years and fertility was high well into the 30s. By contrast, the 1940 cohort reached its peak fertility at age 24 years and tended to have more children earlier in their lives. The 1950 cohort's fertility was stable between the ages of 21 and 28 years. It is probable that family size of the pre-1941 cohorts was determined largely by the age of marriage and that, within marriage,

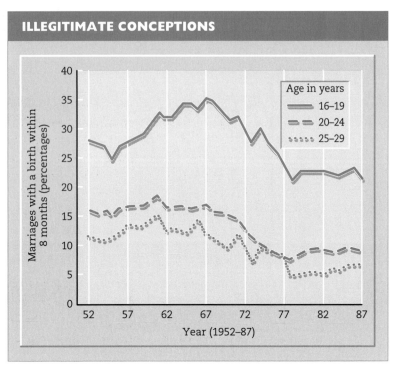

Fig. 10.12 Trends in known illegitimate conceptions in England and Wales.

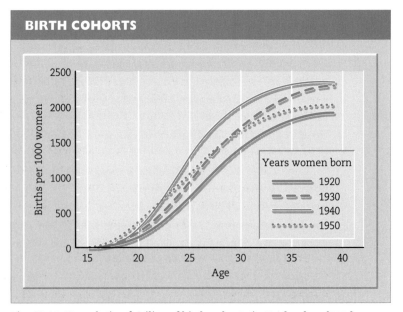

Fig. 10.13 Cumulative fertility of birth cohorts in England and Wales.

conscious control of fertility was haphazard, whilst the post-1941 cohorts married earlier and exercised a more precise conscious control over fertility.

TOTAL-PERIOD FERTILITY RATE

This is a useful measure calculated from summing the age-specific fertility rates and expressing the sum of the rates as the expected number of live births per woman of child bearing age. Thus, in Table 10.1, we can see the UK total-period fertility rate is 1.84 which is below the replacement level of 2.0. In fact, because some children die before they reach reproductive age, the replacement total-period fertility rate is about 2.1 in the UK, and in countries with high infant and child mortality the rate will be even greater.

FETAL LOSS AND INFANT MORTALITY

Fetal and infant survival rates are amongst the most important factors influencing demographic change. Fetal loss during pregnancy occurs in three ways.

FETAL LOSS

- Spontaneous abortion
- Induced abortion
- Stillbirths

In developed countries, 15–25% of known conceptions spontaneously abort. The true rate may be as high as 40%. Sixty per cent of spontaneous abortions have abnormal chromosomes. In the process of demographic transition, changes in spontaneous abortion and stillbirth rates are not significant elements. Induced abortion depends upon individual motivation and it affects age-specific birth rates selectively. In countries where induced abortion is legal, full statistics are published. Figure 10.14 shows the numbers of 'known' conceptions in women aged 16–19 years in England and Wales from 1969 to 1986, and demonstrates the contribution of legal abortion to the fall in birth rate.

Perinatal and infant mortality rates are sometimes used as sensitive indicators of the quality of health services within a country or within a district. This is asserted because some of the causes of perinatal and infant deaths are avoidable by medical intervention.

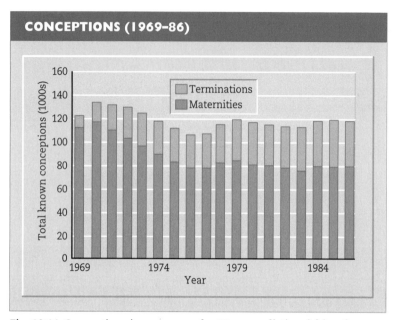

Fig. 10.14 Conceptions in women under 20 years, distinguishing those leading to maternities from those terminated by abortion.

There have been three major studies of perinatal deaths in Britain, in 1946, 1958 and 1970. Cohorts of births were followed up beyond the perinatal period to examine factors related to perinatal mortality and morbidity. They showed that adverse maternal obstetric factors act in a cumulative manner. PMRs are highest in para 3+ women, in women at the end of reproductive life and when the birth interval is less than 12 months or more than 60 months. Conversely, they are lowest in para 1 women, women aged 20–29 years and when the birth interval is 18–35 months. The PMR is higher for illegitimate births than it is for legitimate births, even after account is taken of parity and maternal age. There is a positive social class gradient, i.e. social class V has PMRs greater than social class I. Some social class differences are due to reproductive behaviour. Birth weight is highly correlated with perinatal mortality. The proportion of low birth-weight babies born within a country largely determines its PMR. Also, there is a close correlation between low birth weight and certain maternal factors, for example parity, birth interval and maternal age.

Poor maternal health can also adversely affect PMRs. Important diseases or conditions that have been shown to be associated with high PMR include the following.

FACTORS ASSOCIATED WITH HIGH PMR

- Hypertension
- Poorly controlled diabetes
- Renal disease (which can also decrease fertility)
- Infection (hepatitis B, syphilis, rubella, cytomegalovirus and toxoplasmosis can cause fetal abnormalities)
- Severe malnutrition
- Smoking
- Alcohol can cause fetal alcohol syndrome (intra-uterine growth retardation, developmental delay and spontaneous abortion)

Thus, while a large proportion of fetal and perinatal mortality is difficult to prevent, much can be done to reduce rates by appropriate antenatal and postnatal care and advice.

SUMMARY

- Every industrialized nation has low mortality compared with non-industrialized countries. Further substantial decline in mortality in industrialized countries is unlikely because the major causes of death are associated with old age.
- There is great potential for further substantial reduction in mortality in Asia, Africa and Latin America. This will be achieved by control of the major infective diseases, especially gastrointestinal and respiratory infections in children.
- The principal factors acting against any quick reduction in mortality in developing countries are malnutrition, illiteracy and poverty.
- Industrialization is inversely related to changes in fertility. Four explanations for this can be adduced as follows.
  - In urban societies children are not an economic asset.
  - As the infant death rate declines, the proportion of children who survive to adulthood increases and the number of births required to attain a desired family size is smaller.
  - In urban societies, there are greater opportunities for women outside the domestic environment, and being committed to child rearing restricts a woman's activities.
  - In educated societies, the influence of secular rationality is stronger which allows readier acceptance of contraception.

PART 2

Prevention and Control of Disease

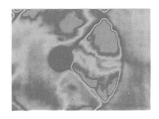

General Principles

INTRODUCTION

The health of the population depends both on the provision of health care for the sick and on public health services to promote health and prevent the spread of disease. Until the middle of the nineteenth century the State accepted little responsibility for the health of the people. The first attempts to improve public health in the UK involved legislation to control the environment. By the beginning of the twentieth century the evident benefits of personal medical care led Lloyd George to introduce insurance-based health care for workers. The majority of health care, however, was still provided privately or through charitable institutions. The State took no major role as a provider of health care in the UK until the inception of the NHS in 1948 which promised access to free health services for all. Today, the Secretary of State for Health is responsible to Parliament for 'promoting and protecting the health of the nation' and the DoH is charged with developing policies in order that 'the health of the nation can be protected, promoted and improved' through the provision of public health as well as personal care services.

Earlier generations tended to accept ill-health and premature death as unavoidable hazards of human existence. People have come to expect a long and healthy life. If illness occurs, it is assumed that modern medicine can, or ought to be able to, restore the sufferer to normal health. These changed expectations of the public have been brought about to a large extent by the publicity given to the more dramatic advances in medical knowledge and treatments and by the evident success of modern medicines in reducing mortality, particularly during infancy and childhood. The public also feel a sense of ownership of the health service and expect ready access to it when needed. Although it is true that during the past 50 years the scope and effectiveness of medical treatments has been extended greatly, it is also true that many of the diseases which commonly affect humans are self-limiting and that medical treatment does little to alter their natural course. Furthermore, few of the diseases that result in death or major disability can be cured. The main impact of modern medicine has tended to be to allow people to live longer and more comfortably with their diseases rather than to die from them or be incapacitated by them. The public often fail to appreciate these facts.

For many of the major diseases, it is both logical and desirable to take steps where possible to prevent their occurrence. Even if a treatment eventually becomes available, a strategy of prevention would usually be more cost effective in improving both public and personal health. In future, it is likely that medical research and practice will be expected to give greater attention to the means whereby health can be promoted and diseases prevented. For some diseases this is already possible and the prospects for further advances in this direction are improving.

Historically, infectious diseases were the major causes of morbidity and mortality, particularly in children and young adults. Their control over the past 150 years owes more to social and economic progress than it does to specific medical intervention. Preventive programmes during this period have included such measures as improvements in sanitation, water supply, the quantity and quality of food, the quality of housing, conditions in the workplace and raised standards of personal hygiene. All of these carry obvious and immediate benefits other than those purely related to health: they make life more comfortable and pleasant with little or no restriction on personal freedom. In fact, most of the changes were at community level and were brought about by legislation rather than requiring action by individuals. This made them comparatively easy to institute. By contrast, some of the more recent advances in the control and prevention of communicable diseases, such as the elimination of diphtheria and poliomyelitis in many countries and the world-wide eradication of smallpox, required mainly medical action (immunization) and thus can rightly be claimed as major medical achievements. The benefits of environmental improvements, as well as of specific immunization, however, will be sustained only by continued vigilance. Much modern preventive medicine is directed to this end. In the past, the presence of a disease in the community served as a constant reminder of its nature and consequences. In societies dependent upon distant memories of serious infectious illness in childhood and once common and often lethal infections such as whooping cough, polio and tuberculosis, continuing public education in the importance of sustaining preventive activities is essential because, with the exception of smallpox, the causal organisms have not been eradicated and the diseases they cause can recur.

The virtual elimination of the older life-threatening infectious diseases has brought the non-infectious illnesses into greater prominence. In modern times, despite the emergence of new infectious disease threats such as legionnaires' disease and HIV, it is cardiovascular disease, malignancies, degenerative conditions (such as arthritis) and other chronic illnesses that occur amongst older people that are the major health problems. There has also been a proportional increase in the importance of accidents. For most of these diseases, the treatments that are available are as unsatisfactory as were the treatments for infectious diseases in the nineteenth century. Moreover, their prevention is more complicated and progress is more difficult to achieve.

The problems of prevention of chronic diseases centre around their natural history, the difficulty in identifying aetiological agents and the fact that many have multiple causes. Moreover, they are generally characterized by having a long latent period between exposure to the aetiological agent and the appearance of symptoms. In many cases, the symptoms have an insidious onset and by the time they are of sufficient severity to cause the affected individual to seek medical attention, irreparable damage has been done. Prevention of these diseases often depends on actions by the individual, rather than passively enjoying improvements in the environment brought about by the actions of others. It demands modification of personal behaviour in such matters as the use of tobacco and alcohol, diet and exercise at a time in life when the risks of contracting the disease in question are seen as remote. It is also a fact that, even for common diseases, the absolute risks for the individual are indeed relatively small. In these circumstances, campaigns to persuade people to change their lifestyle require great skill and patience sustained over long periods of time. These lifestyle changes also need to be complemented by public policies that promote health by, for example, the taxation of tobacco and alcohol products, the subsidizing of food production and the provision of public recreational facilities. These all require a political will to be implemented. Despite the difficulties, prevention remains an important aspiration and progress is being made in some of these diseases (e.g. in reduction of cancer mortality), both by action at a political and community level and by persuading people to change their lifestyle and habits.

The interaction between the social and physical environment and health has also been much more widely recognized in the last 25 years by national and international bodies such as the WHO. It has led to the concept of the promotion of a healthy environment and lifestyle being adopted in a number of cities. Acknowledgement that employment, housing, balanced diets and a social and economic environment that promotes health are all important in improving the quality of people's lives and increasing the length of life has meant that both government and local policies which affect social factors have to take into account the long-term consequences to health.

PRINCIPLES OF PREVENTION

Disease is the result of a harmful interaction between the host (humans), a pathogenic agent and the environment (Fig. 11.1). Agent, host and environment form a dynamic system in which, in the healthy individual, the balance normally favours the host. Thus, if the agent is locally absent or contained, or its capacity to cause disease is matched by the host's protective mechanisms, or the environment inhibits the spread of the agent, health is maintained. Disease or injury occurs when the balance is disturbed, for example owing to changes in the pathogenicity of an agent, changes in environmental conditions that favour the survival and trans-mission of the agent to humans, or the breakdown or absence of human normal defence mechanisms. The control and prevention of disease depends on effective intervention in the relationship between agent, host and environment to ensure that the balance remains in the human's favour, or, if disease does occur, to ensure that its progress is rapidly arrested or reversed or its consequences minimized.

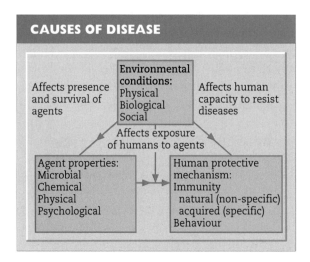

Fig. 11.1 Interactions of agent, host and environment, causing disease.

Useful preventive action does not necessarily require knowledge of the cause of a disease. There are many examples of effective prevention that preceded discovery of the agent or complete understanding of the causal mechanism. For example, in the eighteenth century, Lind demonstrated that during long sea voyages, scurvy in the crews of ships could be prevented by the consumption of adequate amounts of fresh fruit; this was long before vitamin C was discovered. In the nineteenth century, John Snow showed that cholera was transmitted by drinking water polluted by sewage. His findings led to the elimination of cholera by the provision of pure water supplies many decades before the isolation of the causal organism. In this century, Doll and Hill (see Chapter 5) demonstrated that those who stop smoking cigarettes substantially reduce their risk of contracting lung cancer, though the carcinogenic agent in tobacco smoke has yet to be identified. In general, however, a full and accurate understanding of the causes of diseases and of the factors that determine the balance between agent, host and environment is helpful in order to construct appropriately directed preventive and control programmes. Epidemiological studies are used to identify the causal agents and those elements in the environment or in people's behaviour and personal characteristics which are key determinants of the natural history of disease.

INTERVENTION STRATEGIES

Based on the knowledge gained from epidemiological studies three main types of intervention strategy may be adopted.

INTERVENTION STRATEGIES

Strategies related to:
• Agent
• Environment
• Humans

Strategies related to the agent

If the agent can be identified, it may be possible to remove or destroy it at source. For example, by ceasing to use asbestos as an insulating material, the incidence of mesothelioma should be reduced; the control of bovine tuberculosis in humans was achieved by eradication of the disease from milking herds.

Strategies related to the environment

These include attention to general environmental factors such as standards of housing, nutrition, working conditions, water supplies, sewage disposal and the control of environmental pollution. Environmental measures directed at the specific causes of individual diseases are also important and people may be protected from potentially injurious agents by the construction of barriers between them and the source of harm. Examples of such measures include the prevention of transmission of food-borne infection by hygienic food production methods; elimination of vectors, for example action to prevent the spread of malaria or yellow fever by mosquito control; the use of machine guards in industry to reduce the risk of accidents.

Strategies related to humans

There are three strategies involving individuals.
• The enhancement of general or specific resistance to disease, i.e. by improved nutrition or immunization.
• The modification of personal behaviour, i.e. by encouraging people to adopt healthier lifestyles by not smoking, moderating alcohol intake, improving diet, avoiding obesity, exercising regularly, etc.
• The use of screening to detect predisposing conditions or the early stages of disease when action can be taken to prevent its onset or control its progress, for example tuberculin testing for tuberculosis, blood pressure measurement to identify hypertension, or mammography for breast cancer detection.

PREVENTIVE ACTION

Action is usually classified as follows.

ACTION

• Primary prevention: prevents disease starting
• Secondary prevention: detects disease early
• Tertiary prevention: damage limitation

Primary prevention

This aims to prevent a disease process from starting. It often calls for strategies directed at the removal or destruction of agents but can also include environmental control, immunization, health promotion and health education.

Secondary prevention

This aims to detect disease at the earliest possible stage and to institute measures to cure or prevent its further progression. Screening pro-grammes backed by effective interventions are the most important examples of secondary prevention.

Tertiary prevention

This is concerned with 'damage limitation' in people with manifest disease by modifying continuing risk factors such as smoking and by the implementation of effective rehabilitation.

High-risk individual vs population strategy

Where a choice of strategy exists, the planning of a preventive pro-gramme should take account of certain practical considerations. The most desirable approach is one that gives the greatest benefit to the largest number of people. In some instances, this may mean that the most effective strategy is to target high-risk individuals. Such programmes, whilst of benefit to individuals, may do little to reduce the overall burden of disease in a population and sometimes a population-based approach which confers a smaller benefit on a large number of individuals may yield greater dividends. The population strategy has the advantage that there is no need to identify a high-risk group—everyone is targeted. Interventions which are simple and require minimal cooperation from individuals are usually the most successful. Economic factors must also be considered when deciding on the most appropriate intervention strategy. Each of these strategies for prevention is considered in detail in the chapters that follow.

CHAPTER 12

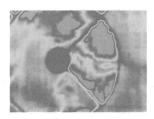

Health Promotion and Health Education

INTRODUCTION

The terms health promotion and health education are sometimes con-fused. Both are strategies aimed at improving the public health, but while the concepts are complementary they are not synonymous.

Health promotion involves the empowerment of the community in improving its health through education, the provision of preventive health services and by improvement of the social, physical and economic environments.

Health education is the empowerment of individuals through increased knowledge and understanding, but does not involve the political advocacy necessary in health promotion.

The health strategies that emerged during the nineteenth century were in many ways similar to those that we now term health promotion. Thus, Medical Officers of Health worked for local authorities with the aim of improving the environment, encouraging healthy public policies, introducing preventive strategies (e.g. sanitation and vacci-nation) and encouraging better health through education. Another step in the development of health promotion was the Peckham Pioneer Health Centre project which began in south London in the 1930s. It provided conventional health care and health education together within an environment which included recreational and sports facilities.

THE NEW PUBLIC HEALTH

More recently, the New Public Health initiative, heralded by the Lalonde Report from Canada (1974), has incorporated health promotion as an integral part of the strategy to improve public health. Lalonde identified four main influences on people's health.

LALONDE'S FOUR HEALTH FACTORS

1 Genetic and biological factors
2 Behavioural and attitudinal factors–the so-called lifestyle factors
3 Environmental factors which include economic, social, cultural and physical factors
4 The organization of health care systems

A growing awareness of the factors that influence health encouraged people with an interest in prevention to involve organizations and institutions not usually primarily concerned with health. This led to the concept of Healthy Cities, which also originated in Canada and was subsequently embraced by the WHO, spreading throughout the world. In the UK, many health promotion initiatives were coordinated under this umbrella, first in Liverpool and later in Bloomsbury, Belfast and Glasgow. At the same time the role of the UK Health Education Council, which was set up in 1968, was expanded to include public policy advice and social and environmental issues in addition to the provision and distribution of health education material.

The key components of health promotion were defined in a charter agreed at the first International Conference on Health Promotion held in Ottawa in 1986. This suggested a definition of health promotion and five key areas for action. The Ottawa Charter stated that:

> Health Promotion is the process of enabling people to increase control over, and to improve, their health. To reach a state of complete physical, mental and social well-being, an individual or group must be able to identify and to realise aspirations, to satisfy needs and to change or cope with the environment. Health is therefore, seen as a resource for everyday life, not the objective of living. Health is a positive concept emphasising social and personal resources, as well as physical capabilities. Therefore, health promotion is not just the responsibility of the health sector, but goes beyond healthy life-styles to well-being.

It also proposed that: 'health promotion should focus on equity in health and reducing differences in health status by ensuring equal opportunities and resources to enable all people to achieve their fullest health potential'. The five areas for health promotion action were as follows.

THE OTTAWA CHARTER

1 Building healthy public policy
2 Create supportive environments
3 Strengthen community action
4 Develop personal skills
5 Re-orientate the health services

Building healthy public policy. To encourage policy makers in organizations and government to place health on their agenda. This may include efforts to identify and remove obstacles to healthy policies so that these become the easier choice.

Create supportive environments. To create living and working conditions that are safe, stimulating, satisfying and enjoyable. To encourage communities to care for each other, and to take responsibility for the conservation of natural resources.

Strengthen community action. To work through effective community action in setting priorities, making decisions, planning strategies and implementing them to achieve better health.

Develop personal skills. To support social and personal development through the provision of information, health education and the development of individual skills.

Re-orientate the health services. To encourage health service providers to look beyond their mandate for clinical and curative services and ensure that health services are aimed at the pursuit of health rather than only the cure of illness.

The principles of the Ottawa Charter were adopted in various ways by many countries throughout the world, but the initial enthusiasm has waned. The UK has adopted health targets in line with 'Health for All by the Year 2000' (see Chapter 18). These targets are aimed primarily at action by the health services without a commitment to changes in public policy. The variable success of the health promotion approach is due to a number of problems. The long interval between the adoption of preventive strategies and measurable improvements in health means that organizations see little short-term return on their investment. The processes of community consultation, health education and altering public policies are time consuming, and are often politically controversial.

It must also be recognized that many health promotion programmes have been initiated without a clear commitment to evaluate their outcomes. Given the limited health budget, it is not acceptable to institute unproved interventions, whether they involve conventional medical treatment or a health promotion programme, unless they are rigorously and scientifically tested.

The emphasis that many politicians and others have placed on personal responsibility for health has been criticized because it ignores the economic and social influences. This can be illustrated by considering smokers who suffer ill health. They are blamed for the outcome of their voluntary action whilst the advertising of tobacco products continues to be permitted and the companies who promote them take no responsibility for the adverse outcome. Similarly, children who grow up in impoverished homes, lacking education and with little hope of employment, have bleak futures and may be unable to respond to the admonition of those from more privileged backgrounds to change their ways. (These issues are discussed in the Black Report referred to on p. 188.)

Another issue relating to the effectiveness of health promotion programmes concerns the dilemma of whether to adopt a population strategy or a targeted strategy. The former involves attempting to achieve health gain through actions involving the whole population while the latter focuses efforts on particular risks associated with specific conditions. Both approaches have their adherents, but scientific evaluation of their comparative effectiveness is needed before one approach or another is taken. An example of a population approach was the North Karelia Community trial, which aimed to reduce the incidence of heart disease in a Finnish community by means of changes in people's diet, smoking habits and exercise compared with a control community. Targeted health promotion campaigns have also been used successfully, for example in the effort to reduce the spread of HIV amongst intravenous drug users by the introduction of needle-exchange schemes.

In the UK many different professional groups and lay organizations are involved in health education and health promotion.

HEALTH PROMOTION IN THE UK

The HEA succeeded the Health Education Council in 1987. It is now a branch of the DoH. The Authority leads and supports the promotion of health in England. It is required to:
• provide information and advice about health directly to the public;
• support organizations, health professionals and other people who provide health education to the public;

• advise the Secretary of State on matters relating to health education. The HEA's strategic objectives are:

• to advise the Secretary of State and other policy makers on the development of health promotion policy and on priorities and targets for health promotion practice;

• to work closely with commissioning organizations to obtain investment in the most effective health promotion interventions aimed at achieving the Health of the Nation targets;

• to enable the implementation of the best in health promotion skills and practice in settings in which people live, work and learn;

• to commission national health promotion programmes which are integrated with local activities and are uniquely suited to direct public education throughout England.

Members of the Board of the Authority are appointed by the Secretary of State for Health for a period not exceeding 4 years. They include leading figures from health, associated professions, the media, education and related fields.

Health care purchasing agencies are charged with improving the health of the population for which they are responsible. Most of their budgets are committed to the provision of personal health services, whether hospital- or primary care-based, but some of their resources are devoted to health promotion. Often this is through health promotion units managed and funded directly by the agency. These units use a combination of health education and community support to target particular issues identified by the purchasing agency. They tend to concentrate on high-profile issues such as cervical cancer, HIV or heart disease.

General practitioners have always given health advice to patients. Their close contact with people means that they are particularly influential within their communities in bringing about change. Purchasing agencies now recognize this contribution and have tried to encourage and coordinate the activities of general practitioners through payments for health promotion. Particular emphasis is placed on the general practitioners' expertise in improving individuals' knowledge and achieving a change in behaviour. The health promotion payments are an example of how primary care doctors have been encouraged to take a preventive rather than an exclusively curative or caring approach in their work.

Voluntary bodies, such as the Royal Society for the Prevention of Accidents, the British Heart Foundation, the Imperial Cancer Research

Fund or environmental groups such as Greenpeace and the Friends of the Earth, are all active in health promotion. Their contribution to the provision of knowledge to individuals, influence on public policy and help in re-orientating the health services is increasingly recognized.

HEALTH PROMOTION PROGRAMMES

There are many different health promotion programmes. Some leading examples of current activities are outlined below.

HEALTH PROMOTION

Target areas are:
* Smoking
* Alcohol
* Nutrition
* Exercise
* Sexuality

Smoking

The UK has a long history of providing information about the dangers of smoking through the campaigns of the HEA, advice from general practitioners and health campaigns in schools.

A Punitive tax on tobacco is one public health policy which has been shown to be effective in reducing smoking. A 10% rise in price has been associated with a 1% reduction in smoking. Banning the sale of cigarettes to children under the age of 16 years and the prohibition of smoking in certain public places are other examples of relevant legislative policies. The banning of advertising has been shown to reduce tobacco consumption, but so far the tobacco lobby has been successful in minimizing legislation against advertising in the UK. The European Union unfortunately continues to subsidize tobacco growing in some member states and it has no agreed policy to reduce the ill effects of tobacco.

Many companies and hospitals have attempted to create healthier environments by the introduction of no-smoking policies. Some have also funded smoking cessation support for their staff. Many cinemas, airlines and restaurants now ban smoking.

Little is done to support voluntary organizations financially in their campaigns against tobacco. A Canadian campaign involving health authorities, Action on Smoking and Health (ASH) and the Canadian Cancer

Society demonstrated the effectiveness of combined action in achieving a ban on tobacco advertising in that country.

One of the goals that general practitioners have been set as part of their health promotion payments involves identifying the number of tobacco smokers within their practice. This is another example of how the health service can begin to move from providing a curative approach to one where prevention and education is the goal.

Alcohol

Doctors have not been good advocates or role models for the prevention of alcohol abuse. The tradition of medical student drinking leads to the development of unhelpful professional and personal attitudes to drink. Restraint in this environment is not easy for a medical student and commonly student habits and attitudes to alcohol are carried over into professional life.

Public policies relating to alcohol include the imposition of excise duties–the UK has among the highest rates in the EU. The historical licensing laws were aimed at reducing alcohol abuse and stemmed from the need to control the gin palaces of the eighteenth and nineteenth centuries, but are now being relaxed. The drink–driving laws have resulted in a considerable reduction in the number of deaths on the roads.

Strategies aimed at creating supportive environments to contain the abuse of alcohol should include offering people healthy choices, for example putting water on the table at mealtimes both in the home and when eating in restaurants. Offering food in pubs and other places where alcohol is served also encourages responsible drinking.

Education includes giving people information about safe drinking levels and publicizing the existence of help agencies. Often, conflicting information about the health benefits of moderate drinking is preferentially heard, perhaps encouraging light drinkers to drink more whilst doing nothing to encourage the heavy drinker to reduce intake.

Nutrition

The subject of nutrition is full of mixed messages due to the paucity of consistent scientific evidence on the health effects of dietary change. In most parts of the world, malnutrition is the greatest threat to health. In the developed world, obesity is the greatest problem. Public policy in the field of nutrition has been scant and poorly coordinated. The Health of the Nation document published by the UK DoH promotes a reduction in the percentage of food energy derived from fat and also aims to reduce the prevalence of obesity. There are differential tax (VAT) rates on some foods, but legislation concerning food is generally aimed at minimizing known hazards rather than supporting nutritional objectives.

Education about diet is widespread and often most effectively undertaken by food manufacturers, for example encouraging the consumption of cereals, and the choice of margarine or vegetable oils rather than animal fats. Whilst a population approach to nutrition is attractive, the use of a targeted approach in certain situations is also valuable. For example, preconception advice for mothers-to-be concerning their intake of folate will reduce the risk of them having a baby with neural tube defect. Perhaps more could be done to improve nutrition through the adoption of nutritional policies. This could be a valuable strategy for schools, hospitals and public dining facilities.

Exercise

The health benefits of exercise are widely recognized and yet its promotion is often uncoordinated. This is one area where public policy could have great influence. Some new towns have been designed with cycle paths and well-lit walkways to encourage healthy options for getting to and from work. Some local authorities have invested in sports facilities and made them available at subsidized rates, but many schools have sold off their sports grounds in the last few years.

Knowledge about the benefits of exercise has increased dramatically over the last two decades. This information is now being passed on by doctors to their patients, and patients are referred to rehabilitation programmes which increasingly emphasize the value of physical fitness. Much of this activity is in the form of tertiary prevention as after a heart attack, although exercise is one example where a population approach as a primary preventive strategy seems to have many attractions.

Sexuality

Improving health through changes in sexual behaviour will come from a reduction in unwanted pregnancies and STDs.

Legislation is in place to protect young people from abuse but will do little to reduce the incidence of unwanted pregnancies. The growing number of pregnancies in those under 16 years and the obvious need for contraception did lead to policy statements by the GMC and BMA about the prescribing of the pill to girls below the age of consent. The

Government has a policy of providing free contraceptive services through general practitioners and family planning services, but ease of access to services has to be complemented by appropriate knowledge and behaviour. This is best encouraged through health education and by encouraging supportive environments. The change in attitude to the advertisement of condoms on television, and their widespread availability through supermarkets and other retail outlets was brought about by a need to promote a change in behaviour to try to reduce the spread of HIV. This has had an effect on other STDs as well as making people more aware of the risks of unwanted pregnancy. This example shows how one health issue cannot always be separated from others.

Some changes in health services seem to happen by accident. Making the oral contraceptive available only on a doctor's prescription placed a clear responsibility on doctors which involved them in their patients' sexual behaviour. General practitioners in particular accepted this responsibility so that now family planning advice is a major part of their work. The medicalization of contraception led doctors to become involved in a number of other initiatives such as cervical screening and well-women clinics. The pill has thus been a very successful influence in re-orientating doctors to providing preventive rather than curative health care.

ETHICS OF HEALTH PROMOTION

The ethics of health promotion can be approached using the four principles often used when considering individual care.

HEALTH PROMOTION ETHICS

- Rights and responsibilities
- Beneficence
- Non-maleficence
- Justice

A key conflict arises between the goals of health promotion and the rights of individuals to personal autonomy. People working in health promotion sometimes seek restrictions on personal behaviour in the interests of the public good. This can lead to conflict with a significant sector of the public who wish to retain their autonomy of decision making. Most agree that where the autonomy of others is threatened such as by drunk drivers on the road, it is reasonable for society to intervene. However, legislating against personal risk-taking is more controversial. There are no laws preventing mountaineering or professional boxing although there is legislation on the use of seat belts which are only of benefit to the individual concerned. Similarly, the use of certain drugs is illegal although they only directly affect the individual user. Thus, the law and public attitudes on these issues are not always consistent.

In relation to beneficence and non-maleficence, in many situations the amount of good or the amount of harm that may arise from many health promotion initiatives is not known. This is not a reason for inaction, but the community is entitled to answers to allow it to make informed decisions. Often the initiative to mount a preventive health programme is undertaken without proper consultation with the community. This is contrary to the philosophy of health promotion, but is often due to ignorance on how to undertake community consultation.

As far as justice is concerned, it could be argued that funds should only be spent when there is a good prospect of benefit to the health of the public. With regard to the targeting of programmes the ethics of a population-based approach must be considered in the context of the needs to reduce the inequities in health between the poor and the rich.

These considerations suggest that all health promotion campaigns should at least be submitted to an ethics committee before being implemented and that a facility should be in place to re-examine the issues as the programme progresses.

CHAPTER 13

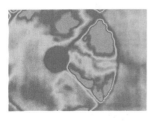

Control of Infectious Diseases

INTRODUCTION

An infectious or communicable disease is an illness caused by the transmission of a specific microbial agent (or its toxic products) to a susceptible host. The agents can be bacteria, viruses or parasites. The majority of microbes are harmless to humans. Some, although not universally pathogenic, are potentially dangerous and may cause disease in unusual circumstances. Caution is needed in attributing a disease to an organism which fortuitously happens to be present as a commensal or contaminant.

There are many factors that determine whether or not biological agents cause disease in a population. They can be broadly divided into the presence of reservoirs of infection, the method of transmission, the susceptibility of the population or its individual members to the organism concerned, and the characteristics of the organism itself.

RESERVOIRS OF INFECTION

A reservoir of infection is the site or sites in which a disease agent normally lives and reproduces. Reservoirs of infection may be classified as human, other biological or environmental.

Human

The human population is the reservoir of infection in diseases such as measles and rubella. Were these organisms to be eliminated from humans, the diseases they cause would be eradicated in the same way that smallpox has been eradicated. However, due to their high infectivity and ease of transmission, these diseases are difficult to eliminate despite the use of mass vaccination programmes. In addition, some infections may be carried by non-symptomatic individuals who may transmit them to others. Asymptomatic carriers are often difficult to identify.

Human carriers are of three types: healthy; convalescent; or chronic.

Healthy carriers are people who are colonized by a potentially pathogenic organism without any detectable illness, for example staphylococcal carriage in the anterior nares or in the axilla, or coliforms in the gut.

Convalescent carriers are people who have recovered from the illness but who continue temporarily to excrete the organism, for example salmonellae in faeces.

Chronic carriers are people who, while remaining clinically well, may carry and excrete organisms continuously or intermittently over a prolonged period, for example typhoid carriers in whom *Salmonella typhi* may remain in the gallbladder for life. Such carriers are a continuing threat to the community long after they recover from the disease.

HIV is of particular interest because the reservoir of infection is human and because there is a prolonged asymptomatic carrier state, followed by a chronic infective state, in symptomatic individuals.

Other biological or environmental

These include:
- animals, for example rabies, malaria, psittacosis and hydatids;
- foodstuffs, for example salmonella and listeria;
- water, for example giardia, schistosomiasis and cholera;
- soil and the environment, for example anthrax, legionella, tetanus.

TRANSMISSION

Infectious diseases can be transmitted by various means and their mode of transmission influences the spread of disease through a community.

Interrupting the transmission of infectious agents is a key strategy for the control of these diseases. Methods of transmission include the following.

DISEASE TRANSMISSION

- Direct contact–touching, kissing or sexual intercourse, e.g. Staphylococcus, Gonococcus and HIV
- Vertical transmission (mother to fetus), e.g. hepatitis B, listeria, HIV, rubella and cytomegalovirus
- Inhalation of droplets containing the infectious agent, e.g. tuberculosis, measles, influenza
- Ingestion of food or water that is contaminated, e.g. salmonella, giardia, Norwalk virus, hepatitis A
- Injection either by human interference or by insects, e.g. malaria, tetanus, hepatitis B and C

Transmission is also affected by the conditions which organisms require for their survival and their life cycle.

TRANSMISSION SURVIVAL

Organisms vary in their capacity to survive in the free state and to withstand adverse environmental conditions, for example heat, cold, dryness, Spore-forming organisms, such as tetanus bacilli which can survive for years in a dormant state, have a major advantage over an organism like the gonococcus which survives for only a very short time outside the human host.

LIFE CYCLE

The life cycle of certain organisms has important consequences in the spread of disease. Organisms such as the malaria parasite which have a complex life cycle requiring a vector are more vulnerable than those with simpler requirements for transmission. In many infections by such organisms, humans are an accidental host.

HOST SUSCEPTIBILITY

Host factors that influence the natural history of infectious diseases include the following.

HOST FACTORS

- Age
- Gender
- Nutrition
- Genetics
- Immunity: natural, acquired and population

Age

The very young and the elderly are more susceptible to infectious diseases than are older children and younger adults.

Gender

There is some evidence that susceptibility to some infections differs with gender. In general, males experience higher age-specific mortality rates than females for most diseases.

Nutrition

The state of nutrition of the host is very important. For example, in developing countries, measles may have a mortality of 5% amongst those who are poorly nourished whilst in the UK the case fatality rate is 0.02%. It is likely that the improvement in nutrition during the nineteenth century was a major reason for the reduction in deaths from communicable diseases at that time.

Genetics

Some individuals appear to have an exceptional susceptibility to infections which is probably inherited. This can be seen in the similar susceptibilities of monozygotic twins and different susceptibilities of dizygotic twins to certain infections. In national or ethnic groups, natural selection over many generations may eventually breed a relatively resistant stock. A good example of this phenomenon is the history of tuberculosis in Europe. During the nineteenth century, the population experienced a high incidence of this disease which, by causing high mortality amongst susceptible young adults, tended to favour the survival through reproductive life of those with higher innate resistance. By contrast, when an infectious disease is first introduced into a community with no recent experience of it, the result can be disastrous. For example, the introduction of measles to the Greenland Eskimos by the American forces during the Second World War caused devastating epidemics with high mortality. Some genetic traits can be an advantage, for example carriers of sickle-cell disease have a positive advantage when infected with malaria.

Immunity

The occurrence of disease in humans depends upon the individual's susceptibility to the agents to which he or she is exposed. Defence mechanisms are: natural and acquired immunity (see Chapter 14) and population (herd) immunity.

POPULATION (HERD) IMMUNITY

The resistance of groups of people to the spread of infection is termed population (or herd) immunity. It depends on the proportion of individuals in the population who are immune. If this is sufficiently high, chains of transmission of the agent cannot be sustained because susceptible people in the group are shielded from exposure to infected people by the immune people around them. The degree of herd immunity which will inhibit spread varies with different infections but is usually less than 100%. It depends on:
• the frequency of new introductions of infection;
• the degree of mixing which affects opportunities for contact between infected and susceptible people;
• the transmissibility of the infection and duration of infectiousness of excreters.

Herd immunity affects the periodicity of epidemics. So long as each case leads to more than one new infection, the incidence of the disease increases and herd immunity rises. When herd immunity reaches a level at which each case causes less than one new infection, incidence declines. As individual immunity wanes or new, susceptible people are introduced to the group, herd immunity again declines and the group is again vulnerable. This was well illustrated by the periodic epidemics of measles every 2–3 years before the introduction of measles vaccination (see Fig. 3.4). Introduction of vaccination programmes lengthens the period between epidemics—the higher the immunization rate, the longer the period. If the antigenic composition of an infectious agent changes or if an agent previously absent from the population is introduced, there is no benefit from herd immunity against that organism and large-scale epidemics may result. For example, antigenic changes of the influenza virus from time to time lead to world-wide pandemics.

CHARACTERISTICS OF THE ORGANISM

The characteristics of the causal organism are also pertinent to the spread of infectious diseases. These include the following.

ORGANISM CHARACTERISTICS

- Infectivity: capacity to multiply in host
- Pathogenicity: capacity to cause disease in host
- Virulence: pathogenicity in a specific host
- Immunogenicity: capacity to induce specific and lasting immunity in host
- Antigenic stability: can induce life-long immunity

Infectivity

The infectivity of an organism is its capacity to multiply in or on the tissues of the host. This varies between microbial species, between individuals and with the route of entry. It may also be affected by the presence of tissue trauma which facilitates the entry of organisms and provides a suitable growth medium.

Pathogenicity

The pathogenicity of an organism is its capacity to cause disease in an infected host (i.e. ratio of number of cases of disease to total number of people infected). In the days before smallpox was eradicated, nearly every infection with smallpox virus in susceptible people caused disease (high pathogenicity), whereas many children infected with polio virus are asymptomatic (low pathogenicity).

Virulence

Virulence is the pathogenicity of an organism in a specific host. Different strains of the same agent may vary in virulence, for example 'wild' strains of measles and polio virus are virulent in humans in contrast to the attenuated strains used in vaccines. The virulence of particular organisms may vary over time, for example the virulence of *Streptococcus pyogenes* appears to have diminished over the last 50 years.

Immunogenicity

Immunogenicity is the capacity of an organism to induce specific and lasting immunity in the host. Some organisms are antigenically more potent than others. Those that invade the blood stream, for example measles virus, are more likely to produce a good immune response than those organisms that only infect surface membranes, for example the gonococcus.

Antigenic stability

Organisms which are antigenically stable or exist in only one antigenic form, for example measles virus, usually induce life-long immunity. If the agent is antigenically unstable, for example influenza virus, or exists in many antigenic forms, for example rhinovirus, humans cannot develop lasting immunity. Environmental conditions, such as those created by the indiscriminate use of antimicrobial drugs, may select out the more virulent and resistant strains of bacteria from among several co-existing variants.

THE ENVIRONMENT AND INFECTION

The environment is the physical, biological and social world external to the individual. Environmental conditions interact in complex ways in facilitating the occurrence and spread of infection in human populations.

For example, climate regulates the natural flora and fauna and the parasites that can survive and be transmitted. If the ambient temperature is warm, the multiplication of salmonellae in contaminated food is accelerated; malaria is transmitted only where the climate favours survival of anopheles mosquitoes.

Similarly, the quality of housing, particularly the facilities for washing and waste disposal, also influences the transmission of infectious diseases and the presence of vectors. When sanitation is poor, epidemics of diseases such as plague, typhus and typhoid can soon re-appear. Improved transportation (whether road, rail or air) between communities has facilitated social intercourse and the spread of infective agents. Infection which spreads from person to person does so more rapidly where there is overcrowding, whether in army barracks, slum tenements or village communal huts.

CONTROL OF INFECTIOUS DISEASES

Some infectious diseases can have serious effects on the health of a population if they are allowed to spread unchecked. They may cause epidemics or the disease may become endemic.* In most western countries, such diseases are notifiable by law to the public health authorities (see p. 90 for list of infectious diseases notifiable in the UK). As many of these diseases are food- or water-borne, the local authority may be partly or wholly responsible for instituting environmental control measures. In other infections, control may be aided by use of vaccines and effective treatment of cases.

Some infectious diseases are endemic in foreign countries and consequently people travelling to and from those countries are susceptible to infection. Measures are required to prevent these diseases being carried back to the travellers' home country.

EPIDEMICS AND OUTBREAKS

The essential characteristic of an epidemic is that it involves a temporary increase in the incidence of a disease, usually circumscribed both in its location and in respect of the groups affected. Rarely, a pandemic of an infectious disease may occur that has a world-wide distribution. The term outbreak is often also used to refer to the localized temporary increase in the incidence of a particular disease. As few as two cases of a disease, associated in time and place, in circumstances where the disease is not a usual occurrence and/or a particular threat are sufficient to constitute an 'outbreak' requiring investigation, for example meningococcal infection.

The pattern of an epidemic depends on the biological properties of the agent, whether or not the environment is favourable to its survival and transmission, and on the immunity of the host population. The course of an epidemic is, therefore, a reflection of time, place and person interaction. Its investigation is an exercise in descriptive epidemiology. Epidemics are usually due to microbial agents although they can arise from other causes, such as chemical poisoning.

* An endemic infection is one that is usually present in a given geographical area or population group at relatively high prevalence and incidence rates in comparison with other areas or populations.

Definitions

Before describing the different types of epidemics and outbreaks and their investigation it is necessary to explain some of the terms used (Fig. 13.1).

Primary or index case: This is the first case (or group of cases) arising from the introduction of an agent into a community.

Secondary cases: People who acquire infection from the primary/index case(s) are called secondary cases.

Incubation period: This is the interval between infection of an individual and the onset of symptoms. This is different for each organism and may vary for the same organism according to such factors as the virulence of the particular strain, the infecting dose and the susceptibility of the host.

Serial interval/generation time: This is the interval between the onset of primary and secondary cases. This interval may be shorter or longer than the incubation period depending on the duration of infectivity of the

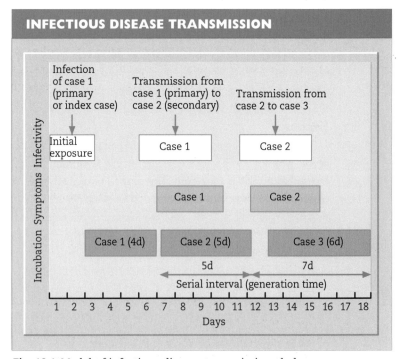

Fig. 13.1 Model of infectious disease transmission. d, days.

primary case, which may start well before and continue for some time after the onset of symptoms. When infection in intermediate cases is sub-clinical, the serial interval may be more prolonged than usual.

Derived infection: This is an infection arising by direct transmission from an infected contact.

Secondary attack rate: This is the number of new cases of a disease arising within one incubation period after the primary case(s). It can be expressed as:

$$\frac{\text{number of derived infections}}{\text{number of susceptible persons in the group at risk}}$$

Types of epidemic

There are two main types of epidemic: common source and propagated.

COMMON SOURCE EPIDEMICS

These epidemics result from the exposure of a group of people to the same source of infection or noxious substance. If exposure is simultaneous for all subjects, an explosive outbreak will occur one incubation period later and the duration of the epidemic will depend upon variation between individuals in the incubation period for the disease. Continuous or intermittent exposure of the population to the causal agent produces a more extended and irregular epidemic curve. The control of such outbreaks depends on the early detection of the cause and its removal at source.

Example: In 1986, there was an outbreak of *Salmonella typhimurium* food poisoning amongst delegates at a medical conference (Fig. 13.2). The vehicle by which the salmonella was transmitted in this instance was contaminated chicken pieces served at a buffet lunch. The resulting gastrointestinal infections caused 196 doctors to report symptoms, of whom 32 were admitted to hospital. Over 1600 doctor-days were lost to the NHS.

Example: In the 1980s there was an outbreak of respiratory disease due to adulterated cooking oil in Spain, initially thought to be due to an infective agent. Twenty thousand people were affected in this epidemic and 430 died. Epidemiological investigation showed that cases were more

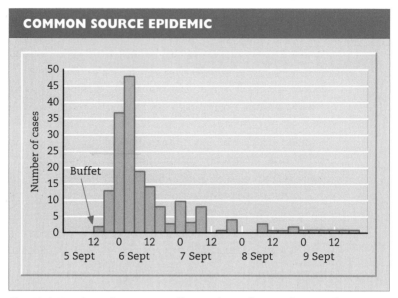

COMMON SOURCE EPIDEMIC

Fig. 13.2 Number of cases according to time of onset. (From Palmer SR, Watkeys JEM, Zamiri I *et al.* *J Roy Coll Phys Lond* 1990; **24(1)**: 26–9.)

common in rural areas around Seville (where the adulterated oil was manufactured) and in poor urban areas. Illicit marketing of the oil was easier in the less closely monitored areas, thus accounting for the difference in the geographical distribution of cases.

PROPAGATED EPIDEMICS

These are due to the transmission of the infectious agent from one person to another, for example measles or whooping cough. In such cases, the epidemic curve usually shows a gradual rise and decline, often with further waves as each successive generation of cases infects a new generation.

The speed at which a propagated outbreak spreads depends on the interaction of a number of factors. These include the opportunity for contact between infected and susceptible people which is itself influenced both by the density of population and by the level of herd immunity. Obviously, person-to-person spread is more likely to occur where large numbers of susceptible people are living in close proximity, particularly if there is a regular supply of new susceptible individuals joining the community, for example nurseries, schools, military camps, etc. Different organisms and different strains of the same organism may vary in their virulence, the speed at which they spread, the carriage rate in a particular community and its duration in individuals.

Remote communities tend to be relatively protected by their isolation from some infections. However, once infection is introduced it is liable to spread with exceptional rapidity because herd immunity is usually low, for example respiratory infections introduced into isolated island communities can cause very high morbidity rates. An epidemic may be initiated from a common source and then continue by secondary spread from person to person.

Example: An outbreak of measles occurred in a primary school (Fig. 13.3). After two index cases in early February, there were two epidemic waves at approximately 10–14-day intervals, i.e. the median incubation period for measles. The outbreak was modified by the fact that many of the children in the school had been vaccinated, including some who contracted the disease. The attack rate in unvaccinated children was high (86%) and showed the typical wave pattern of a propagated epidemic.

The investigation of outbreaks

Most epidemics are public health emergencies and require rapid and coordinated action to identify the cause and to institute effective control measures. It is wise to follow a systematic procedure in the investigation of outbreaks.

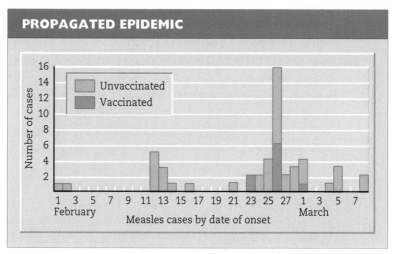

PROPAGATED EPIDEMIC

Fig. 13.3 Measles epidemic in a primary school. (From Graham R, Bellamy S, Richardson HJ. *Commun Dis Rep* 1979: number **16**.)

OUTLINE OF PROCEDURES

The steps described here are not necessarily undertaken in the sequence given. Enquiries usually proceed simultaneously with the analysis of findings and often with interim control measures based on early indications of the likely origin of the outbreak. Not all the steps will be relevant in every outbreak and the questions asked must be adapted to the circumstances. The five main stages in an investigation are shown below.

STAGES IN INVESTIGATION

- Descriptive enquiries into the facts of the outbreak
- Investigate reservoirs and vehicles of infection
- Analysis of the data collected
- Formulation of a causal hypothesis
- Testing its validity in the control of the outbreak

Descriptive enquiries

- Verify the diagnosis by clinical and laboratory investigation of the cases.
- Verify the existence of an epidemic by comparison with previous incidence of the disease in the same population.
- Compile a list of all cases and search for unreported cases by alerting hospitals and general practitioners in the district and neighbouring districts.
- Investigate patients and others who might be involved in the outbreak. Record the personal characteristics of the patients (age, sex, address, etc.) and enquire into shared experiences or activities that could carry risk of exposure to the suspected agent, for example occupation, school attended, recreational activities, consumption of foods, drugs, etc.
- Identify the total population at risk, i.e. all those who may have been exposed to the same hazards as the patients, whether ill or not.
- Ensure that all the clinical and laboratory investigations required to confirm the identity of the infection in patients and to determine the extent of sub-clinical infections are carried out. Phage, serological and other methods of typing of organisms may help to establish the epidemiological association between cases and possible causes (or sources) and to trace the paths of spread of the agent.

Note: The application of other epidemiological techniques such as the use of case–control studies may also be of value in the investigation of outbreaks as a means to confirm the validity of a causal hypothesis. In large outbreaks, investigations can sometimes be confined to random samples of patients and people thought to be at risk.

Investigate reservoirs and vehicles of infection

• *Human.* An epidemic may originate from an individual who has had a minor clinical episode or from a carrier who was ill many years previously. Therefore, a careful history should be taken from all contacts of the patients.

• *Animal.* Enquire about the contacts patients may have had with sick animals or animal products known to harbour the infection concerned.

• *Environment.* Investigate sources of foods consumed by affected individuals and the circumstances of their production, storage, preservation and preparation. Particular attention should be given to looking for situations in which cross-contamination or incubation of organisms could have occurred. Arrange for laboratory examination of food remnants, milk, and water supplies, and other relevant specimens from environmental sources, for example kitchen utensils, drains, etc., and the typing of any organisms that are isolated.

Analysis of the data collected

• Plot of the epidemic curve. This may give some clue to the mode of spread and probable time of initial exposure. For example, an outbreak of *Salmonella napoli* caused by contaminated chocolate bars imported from Italy is shown in Fig. 13.4. Note the relationship between the time distribution of cases and the importation of bars of chocolate.

• Plot the cases on a map. This will detect clustering. The distribution of cases must be examined with reference to that of the population at risk.

• Analyse the incidence rates in different groups. This can be done, for example, for age or occupation. A high rate in a particular group suggests that the cause lies in a common experience of its members. Attack rates must be calculated both in those exposed and in those not exposed to the suspected agent. It should be noted that variations in the biological response to infection may result in clinical attack rates of less than 100% in the exposed population.

• Look for a quantitative relationship. This may exist between the degree of exposure (or dose) and attack rate, for example amount of suspect food consumed or closeness to a source of pollution. For example, in the outbreak of *Salmonella typhimurium* referred to under common source epidemics (p. 157), food histories were obtained from 266 delegates at the suspect meal. Of these guests, 196 reported illness. The food-specific attack rates showed clearly that chicken was the probable vehicle of infection (Table 13.1).

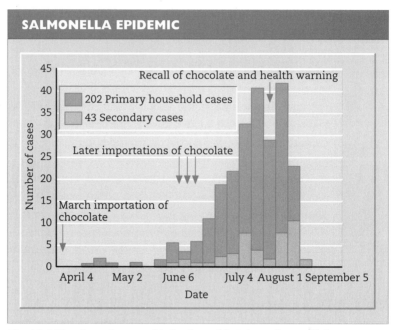

Fig. 13.4 Number of cases of infection with *Salmonella napoli* from chocolate during April–August 1982. (From Roberts JA, Sockett PN, Gill ON. *Br Med J* 1989; **289**: 1227.)

FOOD POISONING ATTACK RATES

	Eaten			Not eaten			
Food	Ill	Total	%	Ill	Total	%	RR
Tuna	70	98	72	127	169	76	0.9
Ham	48	63	77	149	204	73	1.1
Beef	29	46	64	168	221	76	0.8
Salmon	38	46	84	159	221	72	1.2
Egg mayonnaise	67	89	76	130	178	73	1.0
Pate	50	66	76	147	201	74	1.0
Beef sandwiches	10	13	79	187	254	75	1.1
Ham sandwiches	15	20	75	182	247	74	1.0
Chicken	182	213	86	15	54	29	3.0*
Quiche (cheese)	80	108	50	117	159	74	0.7
Quiche (ham)	18	21	86	179	246	73	1.2
Ham and turkey pie	103	137	76	94	130	73	1.0

*$\chi^2 = 70.7$; $p < 0.01$

Table 13.1 Attack rates for delegates eating and not eating specific foods. (From Palmer SR, Watkeys JEM, Zamiri I et al. *J Roy Coll Phys Lond* 1990; **24(1)**: 26–9.)

Formulation of a causal hypothesis

The hypothesis should take account of the following.

FACTORS FOR HYPOTHESIS

- The properties of the agent, its reservoirs and favoured vehicles and also of the nature of the illness it causes
- The probable source and route of transmission. For this purpose the typing of the organisms may be particularly helpful
- Time and duration of exposure of the patients to the agent in relation to the onset of their illness
- Attack rates of the different sub-groups of the population at risk

---

Testing validity in the control of the outbreak

Seek support for the causal hypothesis by further investigation of cases, if necessary, to confirm the proposed explanation of their illness. Carefully designed case–control studies may be very helpful in this. Implement appropriate control measures on the assumption that the hypothesis is correct and monitor their success in reducing the incidence of further cases.

CONTROL OF FOOD-BORNE INFECTION

The most frequently reported notifiable infectious diseases are food poisoning and gastrointestinal infections. They illustrate well some of the biological and environmental factors that are conducive to the occurrence of outbreaks and the approach to their investigation and control outlined above. They also exemplify the complementary roles of the health authorities and local authorities in the investigation and management of an outbreak.

Causes of food poisoning

Food poisoning may be caused by either micro-organisms or chemicals. In the case of microbiological food poisoning, the food may be either the vehicle whereby an agent is transmitted or the growth medium for the organisms. For example:
- salmonellosis may be caused by the organism being transmitted from poultry to humans in eggs;
- staphylococcal food poisoning may arise if during preparation the food becomes infected from a septic lesion in the food handler. If the food is then stored for long enough at a temperature which allows the organism

to multiply, the toxins produced may result in severe symptoms of food poisioning in those who eat it.

The harmful effects of chemicals may arise either from accidental contamination or by the deliberate addition of chemicals to food as preservatives or in order to improve its taste or appearance.

Sources of contamination

Food may become polluted or infected at any stage during its production, manufacture and processing, distribution or preparation for consumption.

PRODUCTION

Salmonellosis usually owes its orgin to the infection of livestock through their food or by cross-infection within herds or poultry flocks.

MANUFACTURE AND PROCESSING

In 1964 an outbreak of typhoid in Aberdeen was caused by corned beef which had probably become contaminated by use of polluted water to cool cans which had defective seals. The 'Epping Jaundice' outbreak in 1965 was the result of eating bread and cakes that were made from a sack of flour that had been chemically contaminated during transit.

STORAGE AND DISTRIBUTION

Outbreaks of food poisoning due to a variety of agents have occurred because butchers, dairies and ice-cream vendors have paid insufficient attention to hygiene when storing and selling their products.

PREPARATION FOR CONSUMPTION

In domestic households and in catering establishments, poor techinque, particularly in relation to avoiding contact between raw and cooked meats, inadequate thawing of frozen foods, insufficient cooking and the subsequent careful control of temperature during storage and serving, together with inadequate attention to cleanliness of premises and equipment may lead to food poisoning, such as that due to *Clostridium perfringens*, staphylococcal toxins, or salmonellae spp.

PREVENTION OF FOOD-BORNE DISEASE

The prevention of food-borne disease depends on correct action by many individuals in the complex chain of production, manufacture and distribution. The main ways in which the safety of food is maintained and good hygienic practice is encouraged are as follows.

Quality of products

There are strict regulations relating to the quality and composition of some foods. This applies particularly to milk and milk products, meat and meat products, shellfish and the use of food additives by manufacturers.

Environmental conditions

Environmental Health Officers of local authorities have extensive powers to inspect all food premises and to sample foods. If necessary they can prevent their sale. The Food and Drugs Act (1955) and other relevant legislation laid down standards on the construction and cleanliness of food premises and equipment, and on facilities for the storage and protection of food from contamination.

Education of food handlers

However strict the law, the avoidance of food poisoning depends heavily on those who prepare it. They should understand the importance of such matters as personal and kitchen hygiene in the avoidance of contamination or cross-contamination of foods. They should also appreciate the need, for example, to store food in protected containers and to adequately defrost frozen meat and poultry before cooking. The dangers of incubating organisms, especially in made-up meat dishes; and the importance of refrigeration of foods liable to contamination in order to reduce bacterial growth and of the separation of raw meat from foods to be consumed without further cooking must also be constantly stressed.

Roles of CCDC and EHO

Cases of suspected food poisoning should be notified to the CCDC which, with the assistance of Environmental Health Officers, is responsible for their investigation. Outbreaks and single cases of serious infections, such as typhoid, call for immediate investigation and control measures. The results may call for amendment of food production, storage or preparation practices in the establishments concerned to avoid the danger of further episodes. In some cases it may be necessary to invoke legal powers to require replacement of faulty equipment, cleaning and refurbishment, or even closure of offending premises.

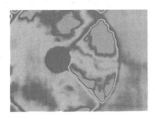

Immunization

INTRODUCTION

Historically, it was common knowledge that people who recovered from some infectious diseases, such as smallpox, rarely contracted that disease again. It was, however, demonstrated by Jenner in 1796 that a person who had been infected with cowpox was uniquely protected against smallpox. This led to the introduction of vaccination, one of the first and most effective of all public health measures. The success of vaccination in eradicating smallpox from the UK and eventually from the world is well known. The isolation of anthrax by Koch in 1876 was quickly followed by Pasteur's attempts to develop attenuated strains that could be used to immunize animals and so protect them against the disease. Pasteur's development of an attenuated rabies virus vaccine that proved to be efficacious in humans was followed by other experiments which showed that dead microbes, or their suitably modified toxic products (toxoids), could also provoke an effective immune response. In 1888, a diphtheria toxoid vaccine was developed. In 1921 Calmette and Guérin developed the BCG vaccine for use against tuberculosis. During the Second World War, tetanus toxoid vaccine came into widespread use whilst an attenuated virus vaccine against yellow fever provided protection for troops serving in the tropics. Today, we have available a great array of vaccines and new or improved vaccines are constantly being developed. The introduction of comprehensive immunization programmes utilizing vaccines against important diseases has done much to reduce mortality and morbidity world-wide, particularly amongst infants and children.

PASSIVE IMMUNIZATION

Whilst most vaccines aim to induce lasting active immunity against specific infections, passive immunization can also be used to give short-term protection against a number of diseases. Passive immunization is the donation to the host of specific antibodies against a particular agent by the injection of blood products derived from immune animals or humans. It is used to give a degree of immediate, though temporary, protection to non-immune patients who have recently been exposed to a potentially dangerous infection. In these circumstances, active immunization is of little benefit because of the delay between administration of vaccine and the production of antibodies in protective amounts.

Products used for passive immunization are immunoglobulins which are now usually derived from the blood of human donors. The historical practice of using animal (usually horse) sera for this purpose has generally been abandoned because of the risk of anaphylaxis. The degree and duration of the protection afforded depends on the amount of antibody present, but significant protection usually lasts no more than 3–6 months. There are two main types of immunoglobulin in use: human normal immunoglobulin and specific immunoglobulin. Human normal immunoglobulin is extracted from the pooled plasma of blood donors. This confers short-term protection against a range of infections that are either endemic or for which immunization is routine practice in the donor population, for example measles and hepatitis A. Specific immunoglobulin is prepared from the serum of individuals who have recently suffered an attack of a specific disease or have recently been actively immunized against the infection. Immunoglobulins of this type are prepared for varicella, tetanus, rabies, hepatitis B and a number of other infections. These products tend to be in short supply and their use is carefully controlled.

Passive immunity to common infections occurs naturally through the transplacental transfer of antibodies from mother to baby. Similarly antibodies are present in breast milk and give babies some protection against relevant infections while they are being breast fed.

ACTIVE IMMUNIZATION

Active immunity to a disease is acquired naturally after recovery from infection with the causal organism.

Artificial active immunity can be induced by the administration of an appropriate vaccine which stimulates the production in the host of specific protective antibodies similar to those induced by natural infection. This provides complete or partial protection, usually lasting at least for a few years and in some cases for life. Active immunization is usually given as a planned procedure. It is designed both to protect individuals against infections to which they may be exposed at some time in the future and to control the spread of infection in the community (population (herd) immunity, see p. 152).

The production of antibodies after the first dose of some types of vaccine tends to be slow and inadequate. Multiple doses at intervals of days or weeks are required to achieve protective levels of antibody. Further re-inforcing doses at intervals may be necessary to maintain immunity in later life. Such doses (or later natural infection) stimulate an antibody response which is always more rapid and usually greater and more durable than the primary response.

TYPES OF VACCINE

Vaccines are of four main types.

VACCINE TYPES

- Inactivated or killed vaccines
- Live vaccines
- Toxoids
- Component vaccines

Inactivated vaccines

These are made from whole organisms which are killed during manufacture. Examples include pertussis, infected polio, typhoid and cholera vaccines.

Live vaccines

These are made from living organisms, which are either the organisms that cause the disease whose virulence has been reduced by attenuation (e.g. oral polio, measles, mumps and rubella vaccines) or organisms of a species antigenically related to the causal agent but which are naturally less virulent (e.g. smallpox (vaccinia) and tuberculosis (BCG) vaccines).

Toxoids

These are produced from bacterial toxins artificially rendered harmless (e.g. diphtheria and tetanus toxoids).

Component vaccines

These contain one or more of the component antigens of the target organism which are necessary to provoke an appropriate protective antibody response. Examples of component vaccines, sometimes called subunit vaccines, include influenza and hepatitis B virus vaccines and *Haemophilus influenzae* type b (Hib) vaccine which is prepared from purified capsular polysaccharide. Acellular pertussis vaccines are also under trial and may replace the whole-cell vaccines as the preferred product.

Vaccines vary in their antigenic potency, i.e. their capacity to induce the formation of protective antibody. This can sometimes be enhanced by the use of adjuvants such as aluminium phosphate or aluminium hydroxide which are included in the adsorbed diphtheria, tetanus, pertussis (DTP) vaccine.

SITE OF VACCINATIONS

The route of administration varies between vaccines. Most are injected, some are given orally. The site of the injection is important for two reasons. Firstly, the antibody response varies depending on whether the injection is given intramuscularly, subcutaneously or intradermally. Secondly, the frequency of adverse effects varies from site to site. Some vaccines, if given too deeply, can cause severe reactions. For example, BCG vaccine must always be given intradermally and should only be given by trained vaccinators. Live polio vaccine is given orally which has the advantage of stimulating local immunity in the intestine and inhibits later colonization (and transmission) of wild polio virus. Most other vaccines are normally given by intramuscular or deep subcutaneous injection. In infants, the recommended sites are the anterolateral aspect of the thigh or upper arm. If the buttock is used, the injection should be into the upper outer quadrant to avoid the risk of sciatic nerve damage.

In order to reduce the number of separate injections, several agents are sometimes incorporated in the same vaccine. For example DTP vaccine includes pertussis vaccine with tetanus and diphtheria toxoids and MMR includes measles, mumps and rubella vaccines. When giving more than one live vaccine it is considered advisable to give them on the same day in different sites (unless an approved combined preparation is used) or to separate them by an interval of not less than 3 weeks to improve the immune response.

SAFETY AND EFFICACY OF VACCINES

No new vaccine is released without extensive safety tests in animals and controlled field trials which establish the level of efficacy and expected nature and frequency of adverse events after vaccination. Careful observance of specific contraindications to each vaccine reduces the risk. Nevertheless, some vaccines frequently give rise to minor reactions, for example local oedema at the injection site, transient fever or rash. Serious systemic reactions, especially neurological conditions, cause great concern but are very rare. To assess their significance, routine surveillance must be maintained. Careful records should be kept of all the vaccinations given, to whom and where, with particulars of the vaccine used. Any serious reactions should be reported at once to the Committee on Safety of Medicines (on a Yellow Card). Likewise, the continued efficacy of a vaccine in controlling a disease should be monitored by the analysis of routine morbidity and mortality reports supported, where appropriate, by microbiological data and antibody surveys. In the UK, these studies are undertaken by the CDSC.

Anaphylaxis

Anaphylactic shock after vaccination is much feared and can be life threatening, but it is a very rare event. Between 1978 and 1989 about 10 cases per year were reported in the UK with no deaths. Around 2 million infant vaccinations are given each year so the probability of a vaccinator encountering a case is very small. Nevertheless, adrenaline and appropriate airways should always be at hand and all doctors and nurses responsible for immunization must be familiar with the management of an anaphylactic reaction.

General contraindications to vaccination

• Immunization should be postponed if the recipient has a current acute or febrile illness.
• Immunization should not be carried out in an individual who has a history of a severe local or general reaction to a preceding dose.
• Live vaccines should not be given to pregnant women.
• Live vaccines should not be given to patients on immunosuppressive treatment or with immunosuppression due to disease.
• Live vaccines should not be given for at least 3 months after a dose of immunoglobulin or a blood transfusion.

False contraindications to vaccination

• Prematurity. Infants who were born prematurely should be vaccinated at the recommended ages, i.e. 2 months, 3 months, etc.
• A previous episode of or contact with the disease concerned, for example measles or whooping cough, is not a contraindication because antibody testing has shown that the clinical diagnosis is frequently incorrect. There is no increased likelihood of complications following vaccination in those who already have natural immunity.
• Mild illness or chronic disease, for example asthma, diabetes.
• Mother or household member pregnant.
• A stable neurological condition.
• Family history of convulsions or adverse reactions.
• History of allergy except hypersensitivity to egg.

Cold chain

Appropriate storage conditions are important, particularly for live vaccines which need to be kept cold. Failure to maintain a 'cold chain' during transport and storage may reduce the efficacy of a vaccine. The most common problem is the storage facilities in many doctors' surgeries, where the constant use of refrigerators for other purposes may mean that the required low temperatures are not maintained.

Consent

Informed consent should be obtained before each vaccination is given. This need not be in writing but parents should understand the risks and benefits of the vaccine their child is being given. Parents should be provided with written information and given opportunities to discuss their concerns.

ROUTINE IMMUNIZATION

The schedule for routine immunization recommended in the UK is shown in Table 14.1. The exact timing of doses is open to variation. While the ages recommended for each vaccine are considered to be

UK IMMUNIZATION SCHEDULE

Vaccine	Dose	Age
DTP	1st	2 months
	2nd	3 months
	3rd	4 months
DT	Booster	5 years
Polio	1st	2 months
	2nd	3 months
	3rd	4 months
	Booster	5 years
Haemophilus influenzae type b	1st	2 months
	2nd	3 months
	3rd	4 months
MMR	1st	12–24 months
	2nd	4 years*
Rubella	Girls if MMR not previously given	10+ years
	Seronegative women	
BCG	1st	10–14 years
Polio and tetanus	Booster	15–18 years (school leaving)

*A further routine dose of MMR at age 4 years has the advantage of boosting immunity in those who responded poorly to the first dose and of protecting those who escaped a first dose at 12–24 months.

Table 14.1 Schedule of routine childhood immunization in the UK.

optimum, it is important to ensure as far as possible that all children are vaccinated even if they present outside the recommended age range, unless there are specific contraindications (see *Immunisation Against Infectious Disease*, HMSO, 1995).

Diphtheria, tetanus, pertussis, and polio vaccines

In order to ensure protection against these diseases as early in infancy as possible, especially pertussis (whooping cough) which is most serious in the early months of life, it is recommended that primary immunization with DTP and OPV should begin at the age of 2 months and be completed by 4 months. Fears about the safety of pertussis vaccine are now largely discounted and any possible risk attached to the vaccine is considered to be slight. Re-inforcing doses of diphtheria/tetanus and OPV should be given at or shortly before school entry. Further doses of tetanus and OPV are required at 15–18 years.

TETANUS

Tetanus or lockjaw has been known to affect humans for centuries. The disease is caused by the circulation of neurotoxins that have been produced by the bacterium *Clostridium tetani*. The toxins cause severe muscle spasms which are extremely painful and may last for a matter of seconds, or continue for many minutes. As well as causing spasm of the jaw muscles (hence its common name), increasingly persistent spasms cause respiratory failure and death. *Clostridium tetani* is found as a commensal in the large bowel of many animal species, including humans. The bacterium can form spores which are able to exist in a dormant state in soil for many decades and when introduced into the body by means of a contaminated penetrating wound may cause local infection with production and release of neurotoxins. A vaccine derived from the tetanus toxin was developed in the 1930s and was administered to millions of soldiers in the Second World War with great success. Today, tetanus vaccination is offered to all infants, with booster doses at 5 years and at school-leaving age. A re-inforcing dose of tetanus vaccine may be required after certain types of high risk injury or burns in individuals who were immunized more than 10 years previously. Where an individual with such an injury has no clear history of having completed a primary course of tetanus immunization, a dose of human anti-tetanus immunoglobulin should be given in a different site at the same time as the first dose of a primary course of active immunization. Those now at greatest risk of tetanus are older women born before routine infant immunization began in 1957 and who were not immunized, as were most men, during compulsory military service.

DIPHTHERIA

Diphtheria is a disease caused by the bacterium *Corynebacterium diphtheriae*. Although often present as a commensal organism of the nose and throat, it can cause pharyngeal inflammation. Certain types of *C. diphtheriae* produce toxins which cause the exudation of the classical pharyngeal membrane covering the fauces. The toxins produced can also cause cardiac failure and death. The bacterium is passed from person to person by direct contact or inhalation of infected droplets and is more common in young people. Thus, children living in overcrowded housing are particularly susceptible. Epidemics of diphtheria were particularly common in the nineteenth and early twentieth century and caused the deaths of large numbers of infants and young children. Prior to the Second World War, there were around 50 000 notifications each year and 3000 deaths despite the fact that a vaccine made from the toxin had been available since the 1920s. The death rate fell dramatically during the war years with the wider use of vaccine, and by 1954 the annual number of deaths was in single figures. Diphtheria is no longer endemic in the UK and the risk of infection derives only from imported cases or in travellers to endemic regions.

PERTUSSIS (WHOOPING COUGH)

Whooping cough was described by Thomas Sydenham in 1670 who called it infantum pertussis (violent cough of children). The Chinese described it as the hundred-days cough. It is caused by the highly infectious bacteria *Bordetella pertussis* and is spread by droplet infection. There is a catarrhal stage for 1–2 weeks before paroxysmal coughing develops. In young infants, the characteristic whoop may not be heard and coughing spasms may be followed by periods of apnoea. Complications of whooping cough include pneumonia, post-tussive vomiting, convulsions, and cerebral anoxia with a risk of brain damage. Most deaths occur in children under 6 months of age.

In the UK in the past, whooping cough epidemics were seen every 3–5 years. Reduced vaccine uptake in the mid 1970s following concerns about the safety of the vaccine led to an increase in the incidence of pertussis, but this has been reversed following much improved vaccine uptake rates and increased population immunity in the last few years (Fig. 14.1).

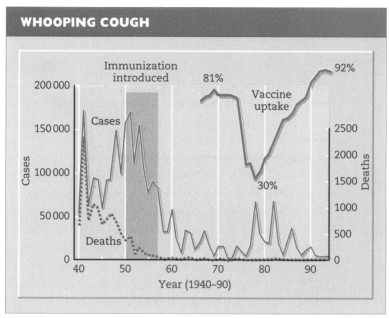

Fig. 14.1 Whooping cough notifications: cases and deaths in England and Wales, 1940–90. (Reproduced with permission of the OPCS (Crown copyright).)

The whooping cough or pertussis vaccine is a component of the DTP (triple) vaccine given at 2, 3 and 4 months. It is in the form of a suspension of killed *Bordetella pertussis* organisms. Concern that the vaccine might cause brain damage has been allayed following the National Childhood Encephalopathy Study (pp. 64–5) which showed that the risk, if any, was extremely small in relation to the risk of disease. Careful adherence to the contraindications to vaccination should further reduce this risk. Children who have had a severe reaction to a previous dose should not have another dose and children with a developing neurological illness should also not be vaccinated.

POLIO

Polio (poliomyelitis) was recognized as a distinct disease in the early nineteenth century and became known as 'infantile paralysis' because it affected mainly infants and young children. The first epidemic was described in Sweden in 1887. Major epidemics occurred in the UK during the late 1940s and early 1950s (Fig. 14.2). The first vaccine developed against polio was inactivated virus (Salk) injected vaccine (IPV) which was introduced for routine immunization in the UK in 1956. It was replaced by the live attenuated virus (Sabin) oral vaccine (OPV) in 1962. Three types of polio virus are included in both the oral and killed vaccines.

Polio is frequently asymptomatic but can cause symptoms which range from aseptic meningitis to severe paralysis and death. Paralysis may be as rare as one in 1000 infections in children and one in 75 in adults. Case fatality in people with paralysis varies from one in 50 in young children to one in 10 in older patients.

The IPV (Salk) vaccine prevents the disease in vaccinated individuals but is less effective than OPV in creating population immunity because it reduces but does not prevent carriage of the virus in the bowel. The OPV (Sabin) vaccine contains live attenuated virus which provides individual protection and also limits carriage and therefore transmission of wild virus. Very rarely the disease has been reported in vaccine recipients or in their non-immune contacts. Vaccine strains of polio virus may be excreted for up to 6 weeks after vaccination. For this reason, while oral vaccine is normally used to immunize children, if there is an immune-deficient person in the same household then IPV should be used. Adults who have not been immunized against polio in childhood should receive a primary course: no adult should be left unprotected against polio. Further re-inforcing doses after that given routinely at 15–18 years are not usually required except for travellers to countries where the disease is epidemic or endemic and for health care workers in contact with

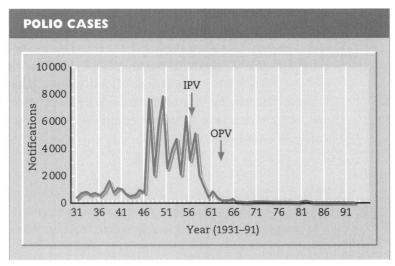

Fig. 14.2 Polio notification in the UK showing the introduction of infected polio vaccine and oral polio vaccine, England and Wales, 1931–92. (Reproduced with permission of the OPCS (Crown copyright).)

possible cases of the disease. Contraindications to polio vaccination include all the standard general contraindications; in addition vaccination should be postponed in patients with vomiting or diarrhoea.

Measles, mumps and rubella vaccine (MMR)

MEASLES

Measles is an acute viral illness which is highly infectious in unvaccinated children. Before the vaccine was introduced in 1968, annual notifications varied from 160000 to 800000 with peaks every 2 years (see Fig. 3.4). Since then, rates have declined with smaller and less frequent epidemics (Fig. 14.3). Complications occur in one in 15 reported cases and include convulsions and encephalitis, otitis media, pneumonia and bronchitis. Measles is thus, potentially, a major cause of acute and chronic ill health in children. Severe illness and death are more common in poorly nourished children and those with chronic conditions, but more than half the deaths occurred in previously healthy children. The vaccine is usually given shortly after the first birthday. Earlier administration is not advised because the presence of maternal antibody may interfere with the active immune response. Unless all infants are immunized and all develop a satisfactory response, there is danger of accumulation of sufficient numbers of susceptible older children to sustain an epidemic. This risk might be reduced by giving all children a booster dose at age 4 years.

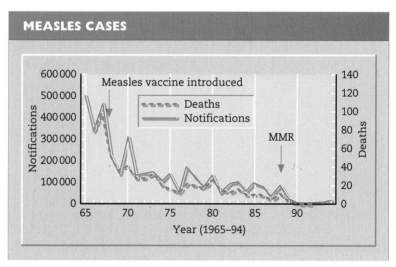

Fig. 14.3 Measles notifications and deaths following the introduction of mass immunization for measles in 1968 and measles, mumps and rubella (MMR). (Reproduced with permission of the OPCS (Crown copyright).)

MUMPS

Mumps is a common but not normally serious illness. However, complications including pancreatitis, oophoritis or orchitis, meningitis and encephalitis can occur and justify the use of vaccine to prevent infection.

RUBELLA

Maternal rubella infection in the first 8–10 weeks of pregnancy results in fetal damage in up to 90% of infants and multiple defects are common. The risk of damage declines to about 10–20% by 16 weeks gestation after which fetal damage is rare. Rubella vaccine was introduced in the UK in 1970 and was recommended for all girls aged between 10 and 14 years of age and for non-pregnant seronegative women of child-bearing age. The application of this policy over the years since 1970 has led to a fall in the number of confirmed rubella infections in pregnant women and with this the number of rubella associated terminations of pregnancy. As a consequence, the numbers of children born with congenital rubella syndrome also declined (Fig. 14.4). However, the selective vaccination of only girls and women allowed continued circulation of wild rubella virus

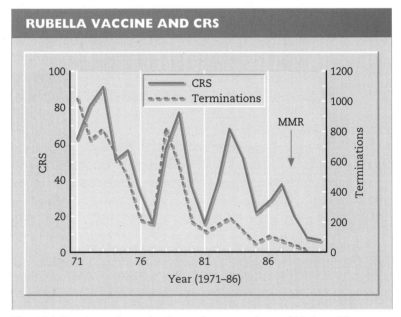

Fig. 14.4 Numbers of terminations of pregnancies and births with congenital rubella syndrome (CRS) following the introduction of vaccine for rubella for girls in 1970 and measles, mumps and rubella (MMR) vaccine for boys and girls in 1988. (Reproduced with permission of the OPCS (Crown copyright).)

in the community with the concomitant risk that a few women who had evaded immunization, or had failed to mount an adequate antibody response to the vaccine, could be exposed to infection in early pregnancy. Since 1988, when MMR vaccine was introduced, both boys and girls have been offered vaccination against measles, mumps and rubella in early childhood. The aim is to eliminate measles, mumps, rubella and congenital rubella syndrome. Consequently, the routine vaccination of girls between the age of 10 and 14 years has now been abandoned but seronegative non-pregnant women of child-bearing age should continue to be given single antigen rubella vaccine.

Tuberculosis vaccine (BCG)

Mycobacterium tuberculosis is present throughout the world including the UK. Other *Mycobacterium* species are also found and occasionally cause disease in humans. *Mycobacterium tuberculosis* was a major cause of morbidity and death in the nineteenth and early twentieth centuries, and there were over 20000 deaths a year still occurring in the UK in the 1940s. It is an organism that usually causes infection of the lung or associated lymph nodes (pulmonary tuberculosis), although it can affect any part of the body (extrapulmonary tuberculosis). Respiratory infection can lead to localized disease, which is short lived and gives immunity to the individual, or it may cause progressive lung disease. Transmission of *M. tuberculosis* is normally by inhalation of air-borne droplets containing bacilli. The infection is more common when people are living in overcrowded conditions. The disease is also more common when the population is poorly nourished or has a high prevalence of chronic diseases.

The death rate in the UK from *M. tuberculosis* has been decreasing steadily since the middle nineteenth century, the reduction being due principally to improved nutrition and living conditions. The advent of effective drug treatment and the widespread use of BCG vaccination accelerated the reduction (see p. 22). Notifications of new cases of tuberculosis reached a low point in 1987. Since then there has been a small rise in the number of new cases (in 1992 there were 5798 notifications) whilst the number of deaths each year is about 400.

Discovered in 1921, BCG vaccination was not introduced into general use in the UK until 1953. The routine use of BCG is controversial. Studies in different countries have produced conflicting evidence of efficacy, the reasons for which are not clear. As a result, whilst it is accepted for routine use in some countries, others have not regarded its benefits as proven and in some, where the incidence of tuberculosis has declined to the extent that it is no longer seen as cost effective, it has been discontinued.

In the UK, BCG vaccine is given as a routine to schoolchildren at age 10–14 years. It is also recommended for tuberculin-negative people in the following categories.

• Contacts of cases known to be suffering from active respiratory tuberculosis.

• Infants and children of immigrants in whose communities there is a high incidence of tuberculosis, who for this purpose may be regarded as contacts. (New-born babies who are contacts need not be tested for tuberculin sensitivity but should be vaccinated without delay.)

• Health service staff. This category should include medical students, doctors, nurses and any other staff who may come into contact with patients or infected specimens from them. It is particularly important to test staff working in maternity and paediatric departments. The vaccine should not be given to tuberculin test-positive people because of the risk of severe reactions.

Haemophilus influenzae **type b**

Haemophilus influenzae is a common bacterium which has a number of antigenic types. It is the *H. influenzae* type b (Hib) which is the cause of nearly all invasive and life-threatening infections, particularly in children under the age of 5 years. It is a major cause of meningitis, with a case fatality rate of around 5%, and also causes life-threatening epiglottitis in young children. The Hib vaccine, first produced in the 1970s, contains purified capsular polysaccharide conjugated to a protein. In 1992, routine immunization with three doses given at 2, 3 and 4 months of age was introduced in the UK. In addition, a 'catch-up' programme was arranged for children up to the age of 4 years. Since then there has been a rapid reduction in morbidity due to this important pathogen (Fig. 14.5).

'HEALTH OF THE NATION' AND WHO IMMUNIZATION TARGETS

The WHO 'Health for All by the Year 2000' targets announced by the European Office stated that: 'By the year 2000 there should be no indigenous poliomyelitis, neonatal tetanus, diphtheria, measles or con-genital rubella syndrome in the European Region.'

The DoH in the UK supported this target and also included mumps and pertussis. To help achieve this, in 1985 the Government set a

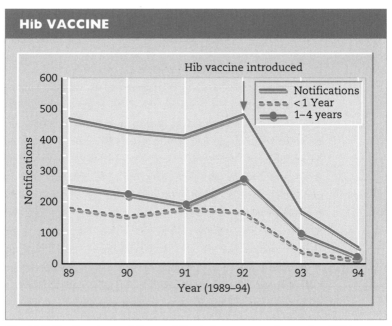

Fig. 14.5 Notifications of *Haemophilus influenzae* type b vaccine (Hib), 1989–94. (Reproduced with permission of the OPCS (Crown copyright).)

national target of 90% immunization rate for children under the age of 2 years. The 'Health of the Nation' programme (1992) revised this to a target of 95% by 1995. Incentives were offered to general practitioners to achieve these targets which generally have been successful. Most UK regions were reporting immunization rates of 90–95% by 1995. However, the targets are more difficult to achieve and sustain in inner cities, and other areas where there is a very mobile population.

The Government also set a target of a 90% reduction in the number of notifications of measles by 1995 compared with around 25 000 notified cases in 1989 (after the introduction of MMR in 1988). By 1994, the number had fallen to around 10 000 cases, but the relatively low historical immunization rates and modest but significant vaccine failure rates left a substantial pool of susceptible individuals. This led to predictions of a large outbreak in 1995. In 1994, the DoH therefore instituted a 'catch-up' programme aimed at school-aged children, to try to improve the population (herd) immunity and to prevent the predicted epidemic. This strategy was effective in the short term but suggests the need to maintain a programme of preschool booster immunization.

OTHER VACCINATIONS

Hepatitis B

Infection with the hepatitis B virus can cause disease ranging from a sub-clinical disturbance of liver function, to acute liver necrosis and death. The virus is transmitted by blood and semen. Some individuals may become chronic carriers, and these individuals are at increased risk of hepatocellular carcinoma. In some countries in South-East Asia the virus is endemic, there are many carriers and hepatocellular carcinoma is a common cause of death. Those infected by vertical transmission from mother to baby, or those infected at a very young age are much more likely to become carriers. In adults, acute liver failure is more common than in children but chronic carriage occurs in only 1% of cases. Hepatitis B vaccine is produced through recombinant DNA techniques. The vaccine is about 90% effective overall; it is slightly less effective in those over 40 years of age. The duration of vaccine-induced immunity is thought to be 3–5 years. It is recommended for doctors, dentists, nurses, midwives, laboratory workers, mortuary technicians, renal dialysis patients, the sexual partners of hepatitis B carriers and infants whose mothers are carriers. Parenteral drug abusers, prostitutes and other sexually promiscuous individuals of both sexes, morticians and embalmers, inmates of long-term custodial institutions, travellers to areas of the world where the disease is endemic and certain members of the police and other emergency services judged to be at high risk may also be considered for vaccination.

Influenza

Influenza is an acute viral respiratory illness that usually occurs in epidemics during winter months. In healthy individuals, it is normally a mild illness, but can cause significant excess mortality in the elderly and other vulnerable groups. Unpredictable changes in the virus surface antigens, which may partially or wholly invalidate immunity acquired from exposure to earlier variants, account for the irregularity of epidemics and, if the antigenic shift is substantial, world-wide pandemics, sometimes with high fatality rates, may occur. There are two main types of influenza virus, A and B, each of which can independently cause epidemics. Killed virus vaccines against both types have been shown to be protective. However, because of the antigenic instability of the influenza virus, the value of the vaccine is variable and unpredictable. Vaccine is prepared from the latest antigenic variants of influenza A and B virus, issued by the WHO. These are for use in the early autumn for people at special risk, such as the elderly (especially those living in residential institutions) and for those suffering from certain chronic diseases including pulmonary, cardiac and renal disease, diabetes and other endocrine disorders and conditions requiring immunosuppressive therapy. The vaccine is not recommended for the control of outbreaks. Live influenza vaccines are still experimental and are not in general use in the UK.

VACCINATION FOR THE TRAVELLER

Overseas travellers are often exposed to infections which they are unlikely to encounter at home. The protection they require depends both on the country to be visited and also on the likelihood of their exposure. Thus, tourists staying in modern urban facilities are at much less risk from many diseases compared to an aid worker or backpacker who may be living or travelling for extensive periods in remote parts where serious infections are endemic and living conditions are poor. Health advice should include both general protective measures and advice on specific vaccinations.

Diseases for which vaccinations are available include those passed via the oral/faecal route (hepatitis A, typhoid, cholera, polio), those spread by inhalation (tuberculosis, meningococcus, influenza), those passed by mosquitoes (yellow fever, Japanese encephalitis) and others such as rabies.

Protection against diseases passed by the oral/faecal route depends principally on good personal hygiene and the avoidance of potentially contaminated food and water.

Typhoid

Vaccination is of value to those who are going to be living in a country where they may have prolonged exposure to potentially hazardous food and water. Both a killed whole-cell vaccine and a live attenuated oral vaccine are now available and will give 70–80% protection. Under conditions of continued or repeated exposure to infection a re-inforcing dose should be given every 3 years.

Cholera

Cholera vaccine gives only limited personal protection (at most 50%) and is not considered to be of value in epidemic situations. Its use is therefore no longer recommended and it is no longer a legal requirement for entry to any country. The principal need in cases of cholera is for adequate rehydration. If properly managed, cholera is rarely life threatening in those who are well nourished.

Hepatitis A

This is probably the most common vaccine-preventable disease contracted by overseas travellers. Those travelling for a short period in high risk areas can be protected by passive immunization using human normal immunoglobulin. Vaccination offers good protection and should be offered to those staying in countries where hepatitis A is widespread. It may be worth testing for antibodies in those over 50 years of age or with a history of jaundice prior to immunization.

Meningococcus

The available vaccine offers protection only against *Neisseria meningitidis* types A and C. Countries where these types are endemic and vaccination is recommended include sub-Saharan Africa, Nepal and northern India.

Yellow fever

This occurs only in parts of Africa and South America. Some countries require an international certificate of vaccination. Avoidance of mosquitoes is the most important protective measure (as with malaria) but immunization with the live virus vaccine obtained from a designated vaccination centre is also of great value. Laboratory workers handling infected material should also be vaccinated.

Rabies

This vaccine is usually given combined with passive immunization with rabies-specific immunoglobulin only to people bitten by a rabid animal or by one thought to be infected. It may also be given prophylactically to those with a high occupational risk or who are working in a country in which rabies is endemic.

Smallpox

With the success of the WHO smallpox eradication programme the vaccine is no longer available or necessary.

Malaria

Each year, some 2000 cases of malaria are reported in the UK in travellers. Most cases arise from failure to take, or poor compliance with, malaria chemoprophylaxis. As yet, there is no effective vaccination against malaria. It is essential for travellers to areas in which the disease is endemic to take appropriate prophylaxis.

CHAPTER 15

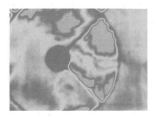

Environmental Health

INTRODUCTION

There has been increasing public concern about the effects that environmental changes are having on the health of the public. This has led to a renewed interest in the real and potential threats from both industrial processes and a range of pressures arising from urbanization and population growth. Strategies for the control and prevention of diseases caused by noxious physical or biological agents are traditionally based on action directed at containing or eliminating the agent. In some circumstances, what is required is a change in behaviour of the general population, for example in trying to reduce traffic pollution in inner cities by encouraging people to use public transport.

Health effects due to environmental conditions can be acute, for example epidemics of respiratory disease brought about by air pollution, or in outbreaks of food-poisoning (see p. 164) or can be long term, for example cancer or fetal abnormalities after exposure to radiation. The long-term effects of adverse environmental influences are often unknown and these are thus considered as potential or unproved risks. Public health doctors have a duty to warn of potential as well as known risks. The design of a rational and effective programme to protect against infectious diseases or to reduce the harmful effects of environmental pollutants requires a clear understanding of the relationship between the agent, the environment and humans in each particular instance. Account must be taken of the properties of the agent which affect its ability to cause disease, the ways in which individuals and populations react to the agent and how the environment can affect the balance between the two directly and indirectly. In addition, the general public want to know not only the relative risk, but are also interested in their absolute risk of disease in order that they may make value judgements about various pollutants and other hazards.

Pollution of the environment increasingly is seen as not only producing physical disease, but also having social and psychological consequences. Thus, although doctors are still concerned with agents such as microbes, chemicals and ionizing radiation which cause physical disease, noise, for example, causing social disruption and psychological stress, is of increasing importance. Global issues such as the destruction of the ozone layer and global warming are also attracting increasing public concern and demand attention.

THE SOCIAL ENVIRONMENT

In many respects, highly developed societies provide a safer environment than those that are less developed. This comes about partly through better environmental sanitation, good housing, clean air, and other physical conditions. Moreover, better education and the provision of better personal and preventive health services lead to an awareness of the importance of a healthy lifestyle. However, economic development also involves industrialization and urbanization. The consequences of these go beyond possible damage to the physical environment. They may lead to disruption of old cultures, weakening of family ties and the creation of communities where support for the less competent members has to be provided by welfare services rather than through an integrated community support system.

Within any society, the poorest tend to be the least healthy. The consequences of poverty, such as poor standards of nutrition, housing, medical services and education, favour high disease rates. The converse also applies: those who suffer from disease, such as the physically and mentally disabled and those with chronic ailments, have the least earning capacity. Persistent disease in an individual often leads to the phenomenon of downward 'social class migration' since the individual is unable to retain the more demanding types of job and is thus forced to live in progressively poorer circumstances in which he or she is exposed to greater environmental hazards and risks of disease. This can give a further downward twist in a cycle of deprivation. Urbanization in general leads to the creation of wealth and in most western countries is reflected in the better health of the majority. However, the large populations who come to live close to industrial installations are often exposed to a variety of related health risks. Again, it is the poorest and most disadvantaged who are forced to live in these unhealthy environments, so worsening the outlook for their health and the health of their children.

Contrary to hopes and expectations, since the inception of the NHS there is little sign that the inequalities in health status between social groups in the UK is decreasing. Indeed, in some cases they may be increasing. The facts were documented in a report, 'Inequalities in Health' (the Black Report) published by HMSO in 1980. The report drew attention to the link between these persistent inequalities and the socio-economic factors influencing the material conditions of life of poorer groups, especially children. Its findings were reviewed, updated and substantially confirmed by Whitehead in 'The Health Divide', published by the Health Education Council in 1987. Further studies have shown that by 1994 the 'divide' was as great as ever.

CAUSES OF POLLUTION

POLLUTION

- Air pollution
- Water pollution
- Sewage and waste disposal
- Ionizing radiation
- Industrial accident

Air pollution

Air pollution in industrial areas arises mainly from combustion of hydrocarbon fuels. The two principal sources are power stations and motor vehicles.

A number of pollutants have been identified as causes of ill effects among exposed individuals and populations. These include the following.
- Sulphur dioxide from the burning of coal or heavy oils. These were the principal sources of the historic London smogs.
- Suspended particulate matter. This can be identified through filtration methods and is produced by both vehicle exhaust fumes (mainly diesel) and industrial processes.
- Lead from petrol fumes has been of concern for some years leading to the wider use of unleaded petrol in some countries and prohibition of leaded fuel in others.

- Hydrocarbons in the atmosphere come from both vehicle exhausts and industrial processes. The potential carcinogenic action of the complex hydrocarbons that replaced lead in petrol is now causing concern.

WEATHER CONDITIONS

Occasionally, weather conditions arise in which there is temperature inversion, i.e. a warm air blanket covering a layer of cold air at ground level. In cities, this leads to the trapping and rapid accumulation of pollutants known as 'smog'. Such high concentrations of pollutants can cause epidemics of respiratory disease.

ACUTE HEALTH EFFECTS

A dramatic example of the acute effects of air pollution was the infamous 'smog' in London in December 1952 (Fig. 15.1) when it was estimated that the fog was responsible for the deaths of 3500–4000 people. This led directly to the passing of the Clean Air Act (1956). This Act empowered local authorities to establish smoke-control areas. As a result, air pollution by smoke declined rapidly in the UK (Fig. 15.2). The benefit was seen when, in December 1962, London again experienced atmospheric conditions similar to those in 1952 (temperature inversion). The excess number of deaths on this occasion was about 700.

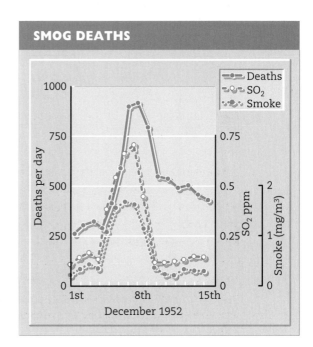

Fig. 15.1 Death and pollution levels in the London fog of December, 1952. (From *Reports of Public Health Medicine Subject 95*. HMSO, London, 1954.)

LONG-TERM HEALTH EFFECTS

The long-term damage to health created by air pollution is difficult to separate from the harmful effects of other factors such as tobacco smoking, but acute and chronic chest illnesses are more common in children and in older people living in areas with persistently high levels of pollution.

More recently, the contribution of the burning of fossil fuels, especially in power stations, to the phenomenon of 'acid rain' with its destructive effects on the forests of central and northern Europe, has been high-lighted. This and the damage to the earth's ozone layer caused by the use of chlorofluorocarbons as propellants in aerosols and as coolants in refrigerators and freezers have become matters of grave concern to ecologists.

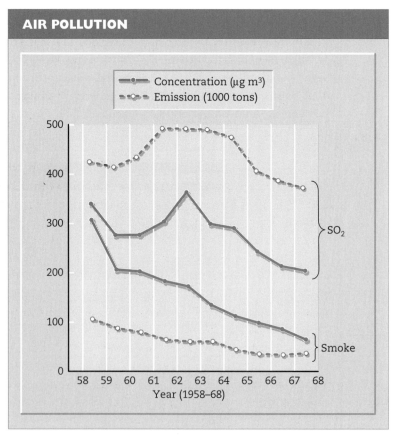

Fig. 15.2 Changes in the emission of smoke and sulphur dioxide and their concentrations in London air, 1958–68.

STRATEGIES FOR CONTROL

As mentioned above, the Clean Air Act of 1956 has had a major impact in the UK in reducing air pollution from the burning of fossil fuels. Monitoring of the emissions from power stations and industrial factories to ensure they comply with the law is the responsibility of Environmental Health Officers employed by local authorities.

The strategy to reduce lead in exhaust emissions from vehicles has been encouraged in the UK by the differential application of duty so that unleaded petrol is less heavily taxed and therefore more attractive to car owners. An alternative strategy adopted by some countries is to ban leaded fuel. Despite this, exhaust emissions continue to be a cause for concern. This has led the European Union to require the fitting of catalytic converters to all new cars. The Department of Transport has said vehicles with unacceptable exhaust emissions will not be licensed.

The removal of chlorofluorocarbons from the atmosphere is being achieved by a number of voluntary agreements backed by the influence of powerful environmental groups such as Greenpeace and Friends of the Earth whose activities have encouraged individuals to shun the use of aerosols and refrigerators which contain chlorofluorocarbons.

Water pollution

The prevention of water-borne disease rests on the purification and protection of supplies. Adequate and safe water supplies are essential to health. To be safe, drinking water must be free from contamination with both pathogenic micro-organisms and harmful chemicals. The main infections spread particularly by water are cholera, typhoid and dysentery. These are due to the contamination of water supplies by human excreta. In countries with modern systems of sewage disposal and domestic water supply, spread by this route is extremely rare.

Storage assists the purification of water by sedimentation of suspended matter and by biological action. It is further purified by filtration through sand or chemical filters. Finally, it is sterilized by chlorination which oxidizes organic matter and kills any remaining micro-organisms. The dose of chlorine is controlled in order to maintain a small residual amount of free chlorine in the public supply. The water is then distributed through a closed system of pipes and service reservoirs. Its purity is monitored by regular sampling at various points in the distribution system.

CHEMICAL POLLUTION

Chemical pollution of water may arise from the discharge of effluents from factories into rivers and streams and also from the use of pesticides and fertilizers by farmers in water catchment areas. A classic example of industrial pollution of water occured in Minimata Bay in Japan in the 1950s. In this instance, pollution with mercury led to contamination of fish with over 100 deaths in humans, paralysis of many hundreds of others and the deaths of thousands of domestic animals.

Generally in the UK, monitoring by the water authorities prevents chemical pollutants reaching a level that is harmful. The protection of water supplies is effected through legislation that prevents individuals and companies from polluting water sources through the discharge of industrial wastes. This has been strengthened by European Union legislation, although loopholes still occur. For example, in Hull the river estuary has been redesignated as coastline and so does not need to abide by the European Union regulations relating to discharge into rivers. The prevention of run-off of nitrates, fertilizers and pesticides from farm land is a problem which may require action. Problems have also arisen in some special circumstances. For instance, the addition of alum to water supplies in order to make the water clearer can lead to problems for people on renal dialysis, as the aluminium salts become concentrated and can cause encephalopathy in such patients.

FLUORIDATION

Where the natural fluoride content of water is high the prevalence of dental caries is substantially less than in low fluoride areas. Controlled experiments have shown that this natural benefit can be obtained by artificial fluoridation of water supplies to a level of 1 ppm. Maximum protection is achieved when fluoridated water is consumed throughout the years of tooth development and this benefit is maintained into adult life. Objections have been raised to the practice of fluoridation of public water supplies on the grounds that it is an invasion of individual liberty and that it has potential dangers. However, trials have failed to show that at the recommended levels any harm results. Relatively few water authorities fluoridate their supplies but the practice is now actively encouraged by the Health Departments in the UK. Probably the most significant benefit to the population from fluoride has been through the use of fluoride toothpaste, but for those underprivileged children who are not encouraged to clean their teeth, or whose mothers do not ingest extra fluoride during pregnancy, the benefit is lost, and without fluoridated water supplies there is further disadvantage.

Sewage and waste disposal

The provision of an efficient sewage and waste disposal system was the single most important public health measure taken in the nineteenth century. Although this is now taken for granted, it remains central to the protection of food and water supplies, as well as to the maintenance of a clean and safe environment.

SEWAGE TREATMENT

In modern sewage treatment plants, after separation of solids by filtering and sedimentation, the liquid sewage is purified by biological oxidation. The final effluent, which is both clean and safe, is usually discharged into rivers (often to be withdrawn further downstream for water supplies!). Unfortunately, some seaside towns still discharge raw sewage into the sea, sometimes even above low-tide level. This practice leads to offensive pollution of beaches and under certain circumstances may cause a hazard to bathers. Where there is no public sewage disposal system, for example in remote rural areas and on camp-sites, excreta are disposed of by using chemical toilets or septic tanks.

Ionizing radiation

Humans have evolved in an environment bathed in ionizing radiation. Today, most of the ionizing radiation to which a population is exposed still comes from natural sources. Consequently, we are unable to calculate the attributable risk associated with exposure to low levels of ionizing radiation from other sources. However, the ill effects of high doses of exposure are well known. This has led to concerns about the safe levels for both individuals and populations. In addition, the potential risk to the public from nuclear war and industrial and military accidents has led to warnings from concerned physicians. The nuclear accidents at Three Mile Island in 1963 and Chernobyl in 1987, as well as numerous accidents in nuclear powered warships, clearly demonstrated that these fears are well founded.

Ionizing radiation can be in the form of X-rays, gamma rays (electromagnetic radiation) or alpha rays and beta rays (particle radiation). Over 85% of the radiation to which people are exposed in the UK comes from natural sources. Around 12% comes from medical sources and around 1% from nuclear fallout and industrial processes. Individuals can be exposed to very different levels of radiation. Some occupational groups such as miners, nuclear industry workers and radiographers/radiologists may be exposed to much higher amounts of ionizing radiation than the general population.

The acute effects of exposure to high doses of radiation include radiation burns, radiation sickness and death. The long-term effects following exposure to high doses have been shown to include cancer (including lung, bone, thyroid and breast cancer) as well as leukaemia, non-Hodgkin's lymphoma, congenital abnormalities and thyroid disease.

Information about ionizing radiation comes from special events such as by following exposed cohorts from Hiroshima, Nagasaki and Chernobyl or people with occupational exposure. In addition, the exposure of large numbers of patients to high dosages of X-rays has given us information about long-term effects. Examples of medical exposure include 40 000 children who in the 1940s had ring worm treated with X-rays to their scalp until their hair fell out, and tuberculosis patients who had large numbers of chest X-rays. Both groups showed an excess risk of death from cancer.

Nowadays in the UK, physicians are interested in the effects of ionizing radiation on the general population, on people living near nuclear power installations or weapon factories and those at risk due to their occupation. A cluster of cases of leukaemia and non-Hodgkin's lymphoma around the nuclear power installation at Sellafield generated particular interest although no satisfactory causal explanation has been found. The cluster has been investigated using both a case–control study and a cohort study, but despite the high relative risks for those children living within 5 km of Sellafield, and for children whose fathers worked at Sellafield, findings from other studies have not supported ionizing radiation as a causal explanation.

Industrial accidents

The general public are not only at risk from accidents that lead to nuclear radiation exposure but are also at risk from accidents involving the transport or storage of a wide range of chemicals. The accident at Bhopal, in India, involving the release of methyl isocyanate gas caused over 2000 deaths and has led to over 500 000 claims for compensation. This was an example of an industrial conglomerate siting a factory close to a residential population in a developing country. Having suffered the horrors of poisoning from the accident, the local population had neither the medical resources to deal with the disaster, nor the legal resources to seek appropriate compensation for the accident. Smaller-scale accidents happen frequently around the world and threaten local communities.

Prevention in these circumstances relies not only on high standards in the workplace but also depends on sensible planning strategies which site hazardous industrial processes away from residential populations.

GLOBAL HEALTH

The concerns of ecologists about the depletion of the ozone layer and acid rain have already been mentioned. In addition, the increasing proportion of carbon dioxide in the atmosphere seems to be leading to an increase in the global temperature which potentially could cause melting of the polar ice caps and a raising of the oceans' levels. This will threaten many island communities. Global warming will also have potential adverse effects on agriculture which may further exacerbate the nutrition problems of many developing countries causing a deterioration in the health of the world population. Global warming and other global issues were the focus of a 1992 WHO conference in Rio de Janeiro which led to an acceptance that action is required by all member countries to reduce the use of fossil fuels, to stop deforestation and for joint action to protect the environment.

CHAPTER 16

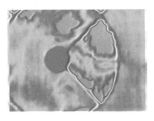

Occupational Health

INTRODUCTION

Occupational health is a specialist subject in its own right, but the activities of occupational physicians overlap significantly with public health. An important part of their work concerns the clinical management of diseases and accidents related to occupations. However, they are also concerned with disease and accident prevention and with the promotion of the health of workers. The principles governing these activities are the same as those that govern the work of public health physicians. Conversely, public health doctors need to understand the ways in which employment influences health and how occupational health services operate in the interests of both workers and the public. Readers are encouraged to consult specialist textbooks on the subject for further details.

More than half the population of the UK spends at least 38 hours a week at work outside their homes. Consequently, the safety of the working environment and its possible adverse effects on health are matters of great significance. However, despite much genuine public concern for safety at work and the existence of extensive legislation aimed at protecting workers, the attention given to the health of workers and the standards of safety that are applied vary widely.

In some diseases attributable to the victim's occupation, the causes are known and specific, and their effects are rapidly apparent. However, most occupational diseases tend to be the result of chronic exposures with long latent periods. In these circumstances, it can be difficult or impossible to differentiate between the causal significance of occupational exposure and other exposures unrelated to the workplace, for example bronchitis amongst steel workers who also smoke. Even when a specific hazard is known and the method of prevention is clear, its application and consequently its effectiveness often depend on persuading employers and employees to act in ways which may reduce profitability and/or earning capacity. Legislation may help, but changing human behaviour in ways that people are disinclined to follow, often a critical element in the prevention of occupational disease, can be difficult.

OCCUPATIONAL HAZARDS

There is a very wide range of potential hazards associated with different occupations. Some are specific dangers, such as those related to handling, ingestion or inhalation of noxious substances (e.g. dusts, fumes, poisons and pathogenic organisms, radiation, excessive noise and accidents with machinery), which can be identified easily. Such physical hazards are usually simple in principle to prevent. Others, like chemical carcinogens with a long latent interval (e.g. the association of nasal cancer with the occupation of furniture making), require careful epidemiological study for their recognition.

It is considerably more difficult to define and deal with numerous other environmental conditions affecting health and efficiency in subtle ways, often more through psychological stress than physical damage. For example, uncomfortably hot or cold surroundings, poor lighting, noisy machinery, repetitive and uninteresting tasks, and excessive fatigue, all tend to be associated with increased accident rates, sickness absence and staff turnover, as well as with reduced productivity. Mental health also is affected by such factors as job satisfaction, boredom, degree of isolation and stressful relationships with colleagues.

PRINCIPLES OF PREVENTION OF ILL HEALTH RELATED TO OCCUPATION

Primary responsibility for safe working conditions rests with the employer. Preventive action which depends on the worker tends to be less successful. There are three possible strategies.

STRATEGIES FOR OCCUPATIONAL HEALTH

- Substitute safe for harmful working conditions
- Protect workers from the effects of dangers in their environment
- Monitor the concentration of known harmful agents in the working environment and, where applicable, in the tissues of workers

Screening for early detection of disease (see Chapter 17) may be necessary where the other strategies are not practicable or cannot be totally relied on to avert the risk that some workers will develop disease.

Substitution

Where there is a clearly harmful material or process it should, if possible, be replaced by a safe one. For example, asbestos which can cause asbestosis and mesothelioma has been replaced by other insulating materials, and shot-blasting has replaced sand-blasting to prevent silicosis.

Protection

If the agent cannot be completely removed, then the workers should be protected from its dangers.

PROTECTION IN THE WORKPLACE

- Enclosure of machinery or processes
- Segregation of hazardous processes
- Ventilation to reduce toxic exposure
- Lighting and temperature control
- Shielding the worker
- Cleanliness and tidiness
- General conditions of work

ENCLOSURE

Dangerous processes or machinery can be enclosed. For example, processes which involve the use of radioactive substances, toxic chemicals or the production of harmful fumes should be conducted in effectively sealed containers. Similarly, moving parts of machinery should be adequately guarded.

SEGREGATION

If total enclosure is not possible, hazardous processes should be carried out in segregated locations. For example, dangerous pathogens such as rabies, lassa fever and Marburg viruses should be handled only in laboratories with effective security. In this way, the numbers of workers at risk can be restricted to those who are trained in safe practices. In some cases, the duration of exposure of individual workers to harmful agents is limited for their own protection, for example where a risk of significant radiation is involved.

VENTILATION

Where the isolation of processes is impracticable, exposure to toxic fumes and dusts is reduced by efficient exhaust ventilation. Ventilation also reduces the concentration of noxious gases by dilution and thereby reduces the risk of their causing harm.

LIGHTING AND TEMPERATURE

Good lighting and comfortable working temperatures help to reduce accidents and stress on workers.

SHIELDING THE WORKER

It is often not practical to devise totally safe processes and, in this case, it is necessary to shield the worker, for example by the use of protective clothing, respirators, goggles, helmets, ear plugs or barrier creams. Unfortunately, such equipment is often hot and uncomfortable to wear, it restricts movement and sometimes vision, and it slows workers down, thereby tending to reduce their earning capacity, which discourages its use.

CLEANLINESS AND TIDINESS

Cleanliness and tidiness in workshops reduces both the chances of exposure to dangerous substances and the risk of accidents. Similarly, attention to hygiene, washing hands or showering, if indicated, and avoidance of smoking and eating in workplaces are important preventive measures in many situations.

GENERAL WORKING CONDITIONS

General working conditions and associated stress may be almost as important in the genesis of ill health attributable to occupation as physical dangers. Attention should therefore be given to such matters as a comfortable and pleasant environment (e.g. in offices), interest of tasks (e.g. on production lines), limitation of hours of work to avoid excessive fatigue (e.g. for transport drivers) and companionship at work.

Monitoring

In order to reduce the risks of harm to workers by exposure to particular toxic substances, careful monitoring should be practised. This may be either by measurement of the concentration of toxic substances in the environment or by biological observations in workers.

ENVIRONMENTAL MONITORING

Environmental monitoring is applied mainly to air-borne substances. The assumption is made that if environmental concentrations are maintained below a certain level, the risk of harm to exposed workers will be negligible. For this purpose two sets of values called *occupational exposure standards* (OES) have been established for a wide range of toxic substances.

Occupational exposure limits (OEL): These were formerly known as threshold limit values. These are maximum time-weighted average concentrations to which a worker may be exposed during a normal working day. Because of biological variation, an occupational exposure limit cannot ensure safety in all workers, and it is prudent to keep as far below the OEL as is practical.

Maximum exposure limits (MEL): These are concentrations which must not be exceeded at any time.

It should be realized that both indices may be exceeded in local situations which might not be detected by general environmental monitoring. Where this possibility exists, workers should wear personal monitors to measure their individual exposure (e.g. workers exposed to radiation risks).

BIOLOGICAL MONITORING

This is concerned with measurement of the amounts of a toxic substance actually absorbed by the body or the early detection of an adverse effect induced by occupational exposure. Biological monitoring should ideally be used to check the adequacy of other preventive methods. Examples of biological monitoring are: the estimation of blood lead concentrations in workers engaged in processes that involve lead; audiometry in those exposed to high noise intensity; proteinuria for renal tubular function in cadmium workers.

The Employment Medical Advisory Service issues lists of suggested 'biological threshold values' for certain substances. Those workers who exceed these biological thresholds should be removed from the hazardous work environment. The degree of deviation from normal values which can be tolerated before damage occurs is often disputed and probably varies between individuals, but guidelines should be based on the absolute risk in an exposed population as this can be predicted with greater accuracy than individual risk.

OCCUPATIONAL HEALTH SERVICES

Although employers are not required to provide occupational health services, they exist in many large industrial organizations. Sometimes, the service is staffed by doctors; otherwise it is provided by nurses with part-time help from local general practitioners. There are a few group industrial health services which provide small firms with services on a contract basis.

Occupational health services usually provide on-site emergency services for workers who are taken ill or suffer accidents at work, and also provide preventive advice to management and workers. Another function is the conduct of pre-employment and routine medical examinations for certain categories of workers who are exposed to special hazards, some of which are required by law. The value of pre-employment medical examinations is controversial. The main aims are to assess an individual's fitness to undertake the work he or she will do and to provide base-line observations against which to compare the results of future examinations. Some medical examinations are designed to protect the public as much as the worker, for example the examination of faecal samples in water supply workers and food handlers, and the stringent medical examinations required for air crew.

LEGISLATION AND OCCUPATIONAL HEALTH

Legislation governing working conditions has been voluminous and complex, having been built up piecemeal since the industrial revolution. It covers such topics as space, ventilation, lighting, heating and cleanliness in workplaces, guards on machinery, safety appliances, fire regulations, the provision of sanitary and washing accommodation and of first aid facilities, and the medical examination and biological monitoring of workers in certain occupations. Responsibility for supervising the implementation of much of this legislation rested in the past with seven inspectorates set up under various government departments. Of these, the Factory Inspectorate, established in 1833, was the oldest and largest. The old, cumbersome legislation was replaced by the Health and Safety at Work Act (1974), a comprehensive, enabling Act giving wide powers which apply to all workplaces. It affects both employees and employers, includes responsibility for the protection of the general environment from the effects of industrial processes, and requires employers to notify accidents. The work of the Inspectorates, including the Employment Medical Advisory Service, is now the responsibility of the Health and Safety Commission set up under the Act. Since 1974, modifications to the legislation on occupational health have been principally through the introduction of new regulations, for example Control of Substances Hazardous to Health Regulations, 1989 (COSHH), Management of Health and Safety at Work etc. Despite these changes the UK seems to be lagging behind a number of other European countries and failure to implement some recent European Union health and safety directives has led to proceedings against the UK. It is likely that future changes in regulations will bring the UK into line with current practice in the European Union.

EMPLOYMENT MEDICAL ADVISORY SERVICE

This service was formed from the medical branch of the Factory Inspectorate in 1973. Its functions are to advise employers, employees, unions and doctors on all health problems related to work. It is responsible for ensuring that periodic medical examinations are carried out on workers in certain hazardous processes (e.g. lead workers), and on any employee whose health is believed to be in danger because of his work. The service is also responsible for advising school leavers with health problems on choice of employment, advising on disablement resettlement services and providing medical supervision at industrial rehabilitation units.

CHAPTER 17

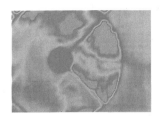

Screening

INTRODUCTION

Screening is the practice of investigating apparently healthy individuals with the object of detecting unrecognized disease or its precursors in order that measures can be taken that will prevent or delay the development of disease or improve the prognosis. The rationale behind use of the screening approach to the prevention of morbidity and mortality is discussed below.

In many diseases, the pathological process is established long before the appearance of the symptoms and signs which alert people to the need to seek medical advice. By this time, the disease process and the consequent damage may be irreversible or difficult to treat. For example, in phenylketonuria (an inborn error of metabolism) the abnormality does not usually declare itself before irreversible brain damage has occurred. This can be averted if the condition is detected in the neonatal period and the affected infant is given a diet low in phenylalanine. In other diseases, patients with signs of disease, for example a woman with a lump in the breast or a person with impaired vision, may fail to consult a doctor because the symptoms are not sufficiently troublesome or because of fear or stoicism or for other reasons. It seems logical to believe that if potentially serious diseases were diagnosed and treated at an early stage many personal disasters may be averted. If so, a programme aimed at their early detection would be a valuable preventive service.

In other diseases it may be possible to intervene at an even earlier stage in their natural history by treating precursor conditions, thereby reducing the risk that pathology will develop. For example, there is evidence that the risk of stroke can be reduced by controlling raised blood pressure, and that the risk of a woman developing invasive carcinoma of the cervix uteri is reduced by the detection and treatment of carcinoma-*in-situ*.

In some circumstances it may be possible to identify individuals who are particularly vulnerable to disease, even though as yet no abnormality exists. Active intervention at this stage may reduce subsequent risk. For example, haemolytic disease of the newborn can be prevented by the administration of anti-D antiserum to the rhesus-negative mother of a rhesus-positive fetus.

Screening for genetic abnormalities is an important recent development. The purpose of this screening is to identify people who are apparently normal but at risk for having affected children, i.e. gene carriers. The carrier individuals are then able to make informed reproductive choices. The incidence of diseases such as Huntington's chorea, fragile X syndrome and cystic fibrosis may be controlled in this way.

Another application of screening is to protect the public health. Some individuals may be infected with an organism and, although they have no symptoms, are capable of transmitting it to others. Such individuals are called healthy carriers. The detection of the organism in such people will be of no benefit to them since they suffer no adverse consequences. However, it is often in the interests of the people with whom they come in contact and the wider community that they should be identified. Ideally once identified they should be treated, but in some circumstances it is not possible to eliminate the organism, for example typhoid carriers. When treatment is not possible, it may be advisable to isolate the affected individuals from situations that may expose others to danger. For example, in an outbreak of penicillin-resistant *Staphylococcus* wound infections on a surgical unit it would be reasonable to screen all the operating theatre and ward staff in an attempt to identify any healthy carriers. Once identified, such carriers would be taken off clinical duties until such time as he or she was proven to be clear of infection.

The use of screening in disease control involves some important assumptions. Some programmes, for example, rest on the assumption that a pathological process can be detected reliably before it is clinically manifest and that, if it is so detected, it can be reversed, arrested, retarded or alleviated more readily than if treatment were delayed until the patient presented with symptoms. For instance, the cervical cytology screening programme depends on two assumptions neither of which has ever been scientifically proven. The first of these is that carcinoma-*in-situ*, the condition which the screening process detects, commonly progresses to invasive carcinoma. The second is that invasive cervical carcinoma is invariably preceded by a phase of carcinoma-*in-situ*. If either of these assumptions is invalid, the rationale of the programme fails. Moreover, it is impossible for obvious ethical reasons to carry out the long-term studies which would be required to test them. Thus, the benefits of some screening programmes are theoretical rather than proven, and in future it will be desirable to test the effectiveness of screening programmes with RCTs *before* their introduction.

Sometimes, the early detection of disease serves only to extend the period of awareness that it is present without improving the prognosis. Furthermore, in any screening programme, cases with a long and rela-tively benign natural history are more likely to be de-tected than those with a rapidly progressive and fatal outcome. The dividends from screen-ing in these circumstances can be disappointing, unless the interval be-tween successive examinations is carefully timed to take account of variations in the natural history of the disease in question.

Before embarking on any screening programme it is necessary to emphasize three further important points.

Ethics. In contrast to clinical practice, which involves the patient asking for the doctor's aid to treat established symptoms, in screening pro-grammes apparently healthy people are invited to present themselves for examination. They have the right to assume that this will benefit them, or at least will do them no harm.

Cost. Screening large numbers of people is expensive and can divert both staff and financial resources from other health services. It is essential, therefore, to evaluate screening programmes adequately before they are introduced and to weigh the potential dividends both for the individuals screened and for the health of the community against the gains from alternative uses of the same resources, the so-called 'opportunity cost'.

Effectiveness. In order to achieve their aim of reducing levels of morbid-ity and/or mortality from a particular disease, screening programmes require a high uptake rate, especially amongst particularly vulnerable groups. This is not always easy to achieve as has been found in cervical cytology screening where the most vulnerable groups—social classes IV and V—have the poorest uptake.

SCREENING PROGRAMMES

There are two approaches to *population screening* programmes. One is to restrict screening to members of identifiable 'high-risk' groups in a population (selective screening) and the other is to attempt to include everyone regardless of the degree of risk (mass screening). Clearly, it is more economical to focus screening programmes on high-risk groups. Efforts can then be concentrated on securing high participation rates in order to maximize the yield of cases in relation to the effort and expense invested. Whole-population screening is indicated only where it is impossible to define high-risk groups with sufficient precision to ensure that they include a high proportion of those likely to develop the disease (sensitivity) and the majority not likely to develop the disease are excluded (specificity). Even with so-called 'mass screening', the programme will normally be restricted to certain broad categories determined, for example, by age, sex, occupation or area of residence. In both selective and mass screening, the programme may be directed to the detection of a specific disease, 'single disease screening', or include a range of tests for a number of different conditions, 'multiphasic screening'.

TYPES OF SCREENING

- Selective screening–test for disease in high-risk group:
  Single disease screening, e.g. chest X-rays for pneumoconiosis
  Multiphasic screening, e.g. antenatal examinations
- Mass screening–with no reference to risk:
  Single disease screening, e.g. cervical screening
  Multiphasic screening, e.g. biochemical profiles on hospital patients
- Opportunistic screening–in general practice

Selective screening

Tests are used to detect a specific disease, or predisposing condition, in people who are known to be at high risk of having, or of developing, the condition.

SINGLE DISEASE SCREENING

Example: Chest X-rays for evidence of pneumoconiosis in coal miners; amniocentesis for detection of chromosomal abnormalities in the fetus in older women.

MULTIPHASIC SCREENING

Example: Antenatal examinations; pre-employment medical examinations in high-risk occupations.

Mass screening

Large numbers of people are tested for the presence of disease or a predisposing condition without specific reference to their individual risk of having or developing the condition.

SINGLE DISEASE SCREENING

Example: Tests for phenylketonuria and congenital dislocation of hip in infancy; cervical cytology for carcinoma-*in-situ*; mammography for breast carcinoma.

MULTIPHASIC SCREENING

Example: Biochemical profiles on hospital patients; routine health 'check up' (well-woman clinics, over-75-year-olds in general practice, pre-retirement groups, etc.).

Opportunistic screening

Some screening only occurs when the opportunity arises, for example blood pressure screening for hypertension in general practice, or cervical smears on women using an oral contraceptive. This is of use because up to 90% of people will see their general practitioner over a 2-year period, so that it is a cost-effective way of reaching a large proportion of the population.

CRITERIA FOR SCREENING PROGRAMMES

Before the introduction and design of a screening programme, certain criteria should be considered (see box, p. 208).

Importance of the disease

Diseases for which a screening programme is proposed should be important in respect of the seriousness of their consequences or their frequency or both. Thus, breast cancer is an important disease because it is both a common cancer and has a high case-fatality rate. Successful intervention will have a significant impact on mortality and morbidity

CRITERIA FOR SCREENING

The disease	Severity and frequency, natural history
The population	Identification of risk groups, attitudes to screening
The test	Sensitivity and specificity of the test, acceptability of the test
The treatment	Effectiveness of early treatment, availability and acceptability of treatment
The evaluation	The cost of the programme, screening participation rates

within a population. Another example is congenital hypothyroidism which is a rare disease but is worth detecting early both because of its serious consequences if untreated and because it is eminently treatable.

Natural history of the disease

The natural history of the disease must be known in order to identify the points at which the disease is potentially detectable by screening and at which active intervention is likely to be effective: this should be before irreversible damage has been done. Ideally there should be a long latent period before overt disease is apparent. Without knowledge of the full natural history from first detection by screening to the adverse out come to be prevented, it is impossible to know what proportion of those screened positive and treated would have progressed to clinical disease.

Population to be screened

Attention should be paid to the way in which individuals are recruited to a screening programme. Ideally all 'at-risk' individuals should be identified and a systematic effort should be made to screen them all. This may be possible where relevant lists exist. For example, all new-born babies are known and can be screened for phenylketonuria. Those who respond to an 'open' invitation to attend for screening tend to come mainly from self-selected 'health conscious' groups who are often at least risk (low-yield groups) but may also attract those who for one reason or another have delayed seeking advice about existing symptoms (high-yield groups).

Frequently, however, it is individuals in highest-risk groups who have the poorest response rates which, unless it can be overcome, limits the potential effectiveness of the programme.

Characteristics of the test

No screening programme is possible without a simple, safe and inexpensive test which can reliably discriminate between those who have a high or low risk of disease. The range of 'normal' findings by the test must be known. It should be quick and easy to use because the object is to test large numbers of people in a minimum time and at a reasonable cost. Unlike clinical practice in which a diagnosis and a decision to adopt a particular treatment is normally based on the history, the findings from physical examination and the results of laboratory investigations, screening is primarily a sorting process which depends on the results of a single test. This imposes particularly heavy demands on the test.

The purpose of screening tests is to divide individuals into two distinct groups: test positive and test negative. However, test positive does not always mean that the individual has the disease or predisposing condition and conversely test negative does not always mean that they are free from the disease or unlikely to contract it. Conventionally, the characteristics of a test are measured in terms of its *sensitivity* and *specificity* (Table 17.1). Sensitivity is the probability that the test will be positive if the disease is truly present: a/a + c. Specificity is the probability that the test will be negative if the disease is truly absent: d/b + d.

In order to measure the sensitivity and specificity of a screening test, it is desirable to conduct follow-up studies over a period of time amongst people who have been assigned to the positive or negative categories by the test but have not been treated. In some diseases, the presumptive evidence of disease in test-positive individuals is so strong, and the

TEST CHARACTERISTICS			
	Disease status		
	Present	Absent	Total
Test positive	a	b	a + b
Test negative	c	d	c + d
Total	a + c	b + d	

Table 17.1 Measurement of test sensitivity and specificity.

potential consequences of failure to offer prompt treatment are so grave, that it may be unethical to conduct such an investigation. However, if a screening programme is initiated without full knowledge of the test characteristics, problems will arise. Although false negatives will become apparent in due course, these diminish the programme's community benefit. Some of the false positives will be identified by subsequent investigations which precede definitive treatment but those that are not so identified and therefore treated will tend to exaggerate the benefits of the programme. They will also waste resources.

The problems for patients of being falsely assigned to the positive category are that they may be subjected unnecessarily to time-consuming, unpleasant and potentially harmful further investigations. Occasionally, they may be submitted to unnecessary and harmful treatments. The false-negative category presents different problems. Clearly, the individuals concerned derive no benefit from the test itself. Furthermore, they may be falsely reassured that they are disease free, however carefully the test results are reported to them, and may delay seeking medical aid when symptoms subsequently appear.

PREDICTIVE VALUES

Knowing the false-positive and false-negative rates we can ascertain the predictive values of a test
• Positive predictive value is the probability of truly having the disease when a screening test is positive: a/a + b
• Negative predictive value is the probability of being disease free when the screening test is negative: d/c + d

---

Acceptability of the test

The acceptability of a test is an important factor in the success of a screening programme. Symptomless patients are less amenable to uncomfortable, time-consuming and potentially harmful investigations than those who are seeking medical aid for a problem or potential problem that they themselves recognize.

Effectiveness of early treatment

There is no value in detecting a disease early unless there is an effective treatment which improves the prognosis compared with treatment at a later stage. Consequently, clinical trials of the proposed intervention are required, particularly because the frequency of spontaneous regression in the early stages of disease is often not known. The reversion of an observation in the presumed pathological range to one in the normal range must not be confused with successful treatment. Furthermore, treatments must be assessed in a group that is similar to that which it is proposed to screen. For example, if it is demonstrated that early treatment of mild hypertension reduces morbidity in a group of men aged 45–54 years, it cannot be assumed that it will benefit men aged 55–64 or 65–74 years who have similar blood pressures, nor that men in the 45–54 age group with higher blood pressures will enjoy the same improvement in prognosis.

Availability and acceptability of treatment

Clearly, there is little point in the early detection of a disease unless the patient is willing to accept and, where appropriate, to sustain treatment at this stage. When a patient has symptoms and believes that medical intervention will bring relief, he or she is more likely to accept the treatment and even endure some side effects. In offering treatment in the absence of symptoms, the doctor is in a difficult position. Long-term treatment for chronic disorders which cause no obvious and immediate disability, for example hypertension, may not always be successful because of non-compliance. This non-compliance may be because of a misunderstanding on the part of the patient, or because of unacceptable side effects or forgetfulness. Forgetfulness is probably the greatest problem as patients have no symptoms to remind them of their condition.

Sometimes, delay in seeking medical aid in the presence of symptoms may be because the patient is fearful of the disease itself or the treatment which he or she thinks may be offered. For example, some women may delay seeking advice about breast lumps because they perceive mastectomy as a more immediate and frightening prospect than the consequences of the disease, or because they see the diagnosis as a deferred but inevitable death sentence. The success of screening programmes for such conditions may also be limited for similar reasons.

Termination of pregnancy following antenatal screening presents a stark example of an intervention being absolutely unacceptable to some women. If a woman would not consider this in any circumstances, screening for fetal abnormality is useless and should not be carried out.

COST OF SCREENING

Health services are increasingly having to recognize that resources of all types are finite. The cost, including both direct and opportunity costs of a screening programme, must therefore be assessed before its introduction. The calculated cost of a screening programme to the health services should include the costs of all the screening tests performed (both manpower and consumables), the cost of further investigations to discriminate between the true and false positives, the total treatment costs of the positive cases, and the total treatment costs of the false negatives. The benefits include the savings on the treatment of cases if they had been allowed to present in the normal way, as well as the social benefits related to potentially lost earnings or the loss of a parent and the 'value' of pain and suffering that would have been incurred. These are difficult to quantify.

It is of course unreasonable to initiate a screening programme unless there are sufficient resources (trained manpower, hospital beds, technical equipment, etc.) to meet the treatment needs identified by the programme.

PARTICIPATION RATES

Many screening programmes are only worthwhile if there is a high acceptance rate amongst those invited to participate. Reasons for low uptake can be that the screening test is not acceptable to many people. For example, cervical screening, especially when carried out by a male doctor, will be avoided by some women. This may show up through ethnic or social class variations in the uptake rate of screening. Other influences on the success of a programme include the level of knowledge concerning the disease being screened for, the manner of the invitation (letters from the person's general practitioner have proved most successful) and the accessibility of the screening venue.

APPROPRIATE INTERVALS FOR SCREENING

The first round of screening in a population (the prevalence screen) will have a higher detection rate and be more cost effective than any subsequent or repeat screening (incidence screen). Judging the most appropriate interval for repeat screening requires detailed research.

There are two important forms of bias that can be introduced into screening programmes.

Lead time bias

This is the apparent lengthening of survival achieved by earlier diagnosis rather than by efficacious intervention. Clearly, early treatment will always increase survival time by at least the length of the interval between the presymptomatic diagnosis and symptomatic recognition: the so-called 'lead time'. To demonstrate that an intervention is effective, age-specific death or illness rates must be improved. Increases in survival time can be very misleading when used in isolation as a measure of effectiveness of a screening programme.

Length bias

Interval screening is more likely to identify slowly progressive cases whose prognosis is significantly better than individuals with aggressive disease. Consequently, cases identified by screening will appear to have a better prognosis than those who have been identified following the appearance of symptoms. In such circumstances, the overall mortality in the population may be unaltered because the screening programme has missed many of the people with aggressive disease.

ETHICS

The wider application of screening in the interests of the public health (whether in an attempt to control the spread of disease or to understand the pathways by which it is spread) raises difficult ethical issues. They are highlighted by the current concern regarding the spread of HIV. It could be argued that routine screening of certain groups might help in both understanding the dynamics of the transmission of HIV and in its control. On the other hand, as there is no effective early treatment for HIV infection many believe that the pursuance of such a policy would re-present an unreasonable and unacceptable intrusion on the privacy of individuals.

Once a decision has been made that the public good justifies unsolicited invitations for screening, then a number of other ethical issues need to be addressed.

People who participate in a screening programme have a right to information concerning the conduct of the programme. They should be aware of the potential disadvantages as well as the expected benefits and they should be free to enter or withdraw without coercion.

Some programmes can cause unnecessary worry to participants particularly if they have a positive test. This is sometimes called the 'labelling effect'. In addition, some individuals, including some who are falsely labelled positive, may suffer harm from either the screening test or subsequent treatment.

Finally, it is necessary to know whether a specific screening programme is the best way to spend scarce resources. This is a matter of judgement that must be based on good information ideally using a cost–benefit analysis which takes into account all the costs and benefits to both the patient and society. Resources spent on a screening programme may mean that less is available for the provision of health care to others.

All of the above ethical questions should be considered by health staff involved in screening programmes whether they be doctors, nurses or managers.

CHAPTER 18

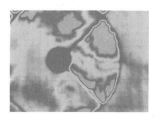

Health Targets

INTRODUCTION

During the past 20 years there has been a shift in emphasis from simply providing access to health care to one of attempting to improve the health of the population. This change has been promoted by the WHO, who in 1975 outlined the concept of 'Health for All by the Year 2000'. 'Health for All' was officially adopted as WHO policy in 1981. It advocated that the pursuit of health, rather than only the cure of disease, should be the aim of health policy makers. In addition, it was suggested that policy makers should strive for more equitable health status both within and between countries. The WHO suggested these goals could best be achieved through promotion of healthy lifestyles, the elimination of preventable diseases and the provision of comprehensive health coverage based on primary health care.

'Health for All' suggested that countries should develop health targets which could be monitored to ensure that the strategies of improved health status and equity were being achieved. The European Regional Office of WHO suggested 38 targets to assist member states in setting their own targets.

Many countries world-wide have adopted the idea of setting national health targets aimed at improving the health of the people. The number and types of target have varied widely depending on local needs and the available resources. For example, New Zealand developed 10 health goals in 1989 whilst the USA adopted 15 key goals and over 200 objectives in 1979.

WHO TARGETS

The 38 targets of 'Health for All' were broken into the following subsets.

Outcome targets for improvements in health, for example:
• eliminating preventable diseases like measles
• reducing mortality from diseases like heart disease and strokes

Process targets for activities needed to make these improvements, for example:
• policies to reduce smoking
• introducing population-based disease screening

Structural targets designed to improve health services management/organization, quality of care, staff training, etc.

The Government of the UK published a strategic policy document entitled 'Health of the Nation' in July 1992 which outlined the Government strategy for improving health in England. Similar documents were produced for other countries in the UK.

'HEALTH OF THE NATION' (1992)

The stated overall aim was: 'to add years to life and to add life to years'. Three criteria governed the selection of the key issues for England:

1 The targets should be major causes of premature death or avoidable ill health
2 Effective interventions should be possible offering significant scope for improvements in health
3 It should be possible to set objectives and targets and monitor progress towards them

The key subjects chosen for action were:
• ischaemic heart disease and stroke;
• cancers;
• mental illness;
• HIV/AIDS and sexual health;
• accidents.

IHD AND STROKE

IHD is due to atheroma of the coronary arteries and is the largest single cause of death amongst men and women in the UK. It accounts for around 26% of all deaths. The incidence of IHD increases with age, and is greater in men than in women (Fig. 18.1). Often in older age groups, the certified cause of death can be arbitrary. Consequently, comparative mortality data usually exclude deaths in people over the age of 70 years.

There has been a steady fall in death rates from IHD in adults in England since the 1970s (Fig. 18.2), and similar reductions have been seen in some other countries such as the USA and Australia. Despite these reductions, comparisons with countries such as France and Japan (which have much lower recorded death rates from IHD (Fig. 18.3)) encourage the belief that further substantial reductions in the incidence of IHD are possible, although some discrepancies may be attributable to differences in recording methods and assignment of causes. Stroke, which is also due to vascular disease and has many of the same underlying causes as IHD, accounts for 12% of deaths. Thus, the scope for making a significant impact on the health of the population if either or both of these causes of death and disability can be reduced is considerable.

The risk of IHD is increased significantly in relation to three key risk factors: smoking, hypertension and cholesterol levels. Around 30% of the adult population smoke. Studies have shown that the relative risk of death from IHD and stroke is increased in smokers compared to non-smokers and increases with the number of cigarettes smoked. Similarly,

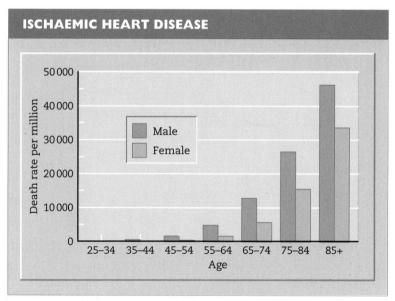

Fig. 18.1 Age-specific death rates for men and women due to IHD. (Reproduced with permission of the OPCS (Crown copyright).)

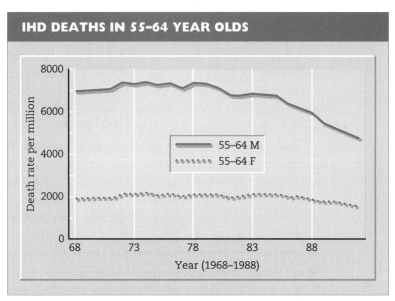

Fig. 18.2 Death rate per million from IHD in adults in England aged 55–64 years. (Reproduced with permission of the OP2CS (Crown copyright).)

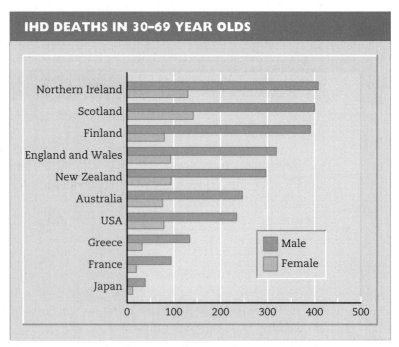

Fig. 18.3 Age-standardized mortality rates (per 100000) in the 30–39 age group, for IHD. (From Uemura and Pisa, *World Health Stat Q,* 1988; **41(3–4)**: 155–78.)

there is a positive correlation between blood pressure and the risk of IHD and stroke. There is also a direct relationship between serum cholesterol and IHD. Related risk factors are obesity, lack of exercise and stress. Effective interventions are available for some of these risk factors, either through appropriate therapeutic intervention or through lifestyle changes. Genetic makeup as indicated by a family history of IHD, and gender are two risk factors that cannot be modified.

The following health targets have been set. These can be considered outcome targets.

• To reduce the death rate for both IHD and stroke in people aged under 65 years by at least 40% by the year 2000.

• To reduce the death rate for IHD in people aged 65–74 years by at least 30% by the year 2000.

• To reduce the death rate for stroke in people aged 65–74 years by at least 40% by the year 2000.

As well as setting outcome targets, targets relating to process were also put in place.

• To reduce the prevalence of cigarette smoking in men and women aged 16 or over to no more than 20% by the year 2000.

• To reduce the average percentage of food energy derived by the population from saturated fats by at least 35% by 2005.

• To reduce the average percentage of food energy derived by the population from total fat by at least 12% by the year 2005.

• To reduce the percentage of men and women aged 16–64 years who are obese by at least 25% for men and 33% for women by 2005.

• To reduce mean systolic blood pressure in the adult population by at least 5 mmHg by 2005.

• To reduce the proportion of men drinking more than 21 units of alcohol per week from 28% in 1990 to 18% by 2005, and the proportion of women drinking more than 14 units of alcohol per week from 11% in 1990 to 7% by 2005.

Work is also being undertaken to try to develop a target related to exercise. The problem with setting such a target is that the present situation as regards the amount of exercise the population currently takes is unknown and difficult to quantify. Data on people's smoking habits, diet, weight and alcohol intake have been obtained from surveys, but continual monitoring is needed before we can be sure that progress towards the set goals is being achieved.

CANCERS

Cancers account for around 25% of the deaths in the UK. There are many types of cancer and the causes of each differ. Health targets concentrate on the most common cancers and those cancers whose prevention would add the most years to life. The four cancers that the Health of the Nation has targeted are lung cancer, breast cancer, cervical cancer and skin cancer.

Lung cancer

Lung cancer is the most common cancer in the western world. In the UK, it is the most common cause of death from cancer in men and the second most common cause in women. The death rate from lung cancer is higher in men and increases with age (Fig. 18.4). The rates of both registrations of new cancers and deaths in women are increasing in contrast to the rates in men which are decreasing (Fig. 18.5). This is related to the changing patterns of smoking in men and women. It is estimated that 80% of lung cancer deaths are caused by smoking. The dangers of passive smoking also need to be considered. It is estimated that non-smokers

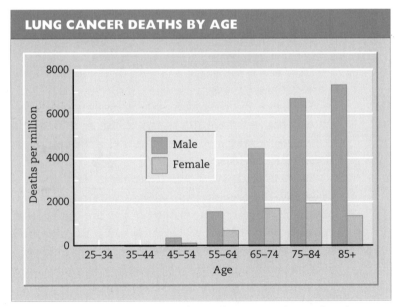

Fig. 18.4 Age-specific death rates for malignant neoplasm of trachea, bronchus and lung in the UK. (Reproduced with permission of the OPCS (Crown copyright).)

LUNG CANCER

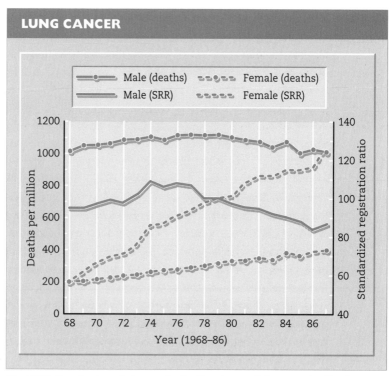

Fig. 18.5 Secular trends in crude death rates and the standardized registration ratio (SRR) of carcinoma of the bronchus for men and women, 1968–87 in England and Wales. (Reproduced with permission of the OPCS (Crown copyright).)

who are regularly exposed to tobacco smoke carry an increased risk of 10–30%. In addition, the difference in the smoking habits of the different social classes is changing resulting in growing inequity in health status amongst the lower classes due to the effects of cigarette smoking. Targets for lung cancer include the following.

TARGETS FOR LUNG CANCER

- To reduce the death rate for lung cancer by at least 30% in men aged under 75 years and 15% in women aged under 75 years by 2010
- To reduce the prevalence of cigarette smoking in men and women aged 16 years and over to no more than 20% by the year 2000
- To reduce the prevalence of smoking among 11–15-years-olds by at least 33% by 1994
- To reduce the consumption of cigarettes by at least 40% by the year 2000

Strategies that have been suggested to help achieve these goals include advice from general practitioners to patients to give up smoking, wider promotion of the dangers of smoking and the use, in appropriate situations, of nicotine replacement therapy.

Breast cancer

Breast cancer causes more deaths in women in England than any other cancer; there are about 12500 deaths per year of which 5000 are in women under the age of 65 years (Fig. 18.6). At least one in 14 women in England develops breast cancer. Rates in other countries differ from those found in the UK, with higher rates in the USA but lower rates in Asian and Hispanic countries. Migrant studies have shown that environmental and lifestyle factors are extremely important in the aetiology of breast cancer. There are many risk factors for breast cancer. It is one of the few cancers where the risk is greater in women from higher social classes (Fig. 18.7). Other risk factors include age at first pregnancy, age at menopause and parity (with nulliparous women being at increased risk). It is unclear whether there is any association between breast cancer and the oral contraceptive pill.

The Health of the Nation target is to reduce the death rate for breast cancer in the population invited for screening by at least 25% by the year 2000. In the UK, women aged 50–64 years are invited to attend breast

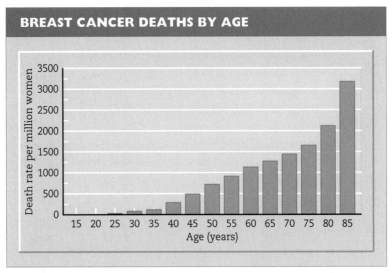

Fig. 18.6 Carcinoma of the female breast. Age-specific death rates in England, 1990. (Reproduced with permission of the OPCS (Crown copyright).)

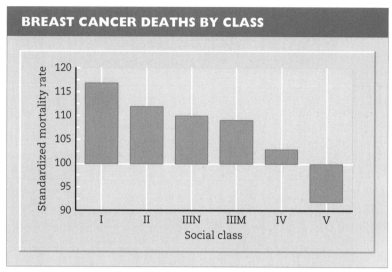

BREAST CANCER DEATHS BY CLASS

Fig. 18.7 Mortality from carcinoma of the female breast in England, by Registrar General's social class. N, non-manual; M, manual.

cancer screening every 3 years. RCTs have shown that when a high proportion of the eligible women attend screening, up to a 30% reduction in deaths can be achieved. Thus, the Health of the Nation strategy to reduce breast cancer deaths involves promotion of the national mammography screening programme.

Cervical cancer

Cancer of the uterine cervix is relatively uncommon. The importance of cervical cancer as a health target relates to the fact that it is the second most common cancer in middle-aged women (after breast cancer), and potentially the outcome can be modified by comprehensive screening and effective treatment of precancerous conditions. There are around 3500 new cases each year and 1500 deaths, i.e. 0.6% of all female deaths. Although the annual number of deaths from cervical cancer has fallen steadily since the 1950s, the number of registrations of cases of invasive cancer each year has remained the same despite the introduction of widespread cervical screening (Fig. 18.8). Cervical cancer is more common in women who become sexually active at a young age, in those with multiple sexual partners and in those whose regular sexual partner has had multiple partners. It has been shown to be associated with the sexual transmission of human papilloma virus, particularly types 16 and 18. There are positive associations with child bearing, with an increased risk

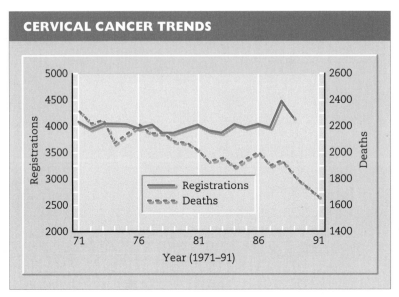

CERVICAL CANCER TRENDS

Registrations ... Registrations

..... Deaths

Year (1971–91)

Fig. **18.8** Registrations of and deaths from cervical cancer. (Reproduced with permission of the OPCS (Crown copyright).)

for those who start having children at a young age, and the risk increases with increasing parity. There has also been shown to be an association with smoking and oral contraceptives. Barrier methods of contraception reduce the risk of cervical cancer.

The Health of the Nation target is to reduce the incidence of invasive cervical cancer by at least 20% by the year 2000. The suggested strategy to achieve this target is to increase the number of women attending for a Pap smear by encouraging all women to register with a general practitioner, and then to respond to the invitation to attend regularly for a cervical smear test.

Skin cancer

There are three main types of skin cancer: basal cell cancers, squamous cell cancers and malignant melanomas. Although melanoma is a relatively rare skin cancer, it is important because it is the most likely to metastasize and is the most likely to cause premature death. There are around 1000 deaths per year in England due to skin cancer. The incidence of malignant melanoma is rising by about 6% per annum (Fig. 18.9). Non-melanotic skin cancers affect over 30 000 people a year in the UK and cause about 400 deaths. Both malignant melanoma and squamous cell carcinoma are associated with excess exposure to ultraviolet radiation

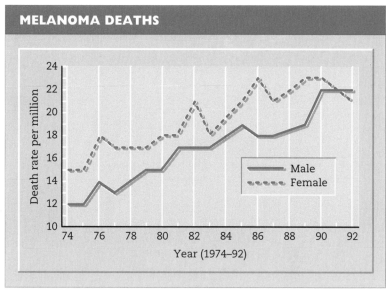

MELANOMA DEATHS

Fig. **18.9** Crude death rate from malignant melanoma 1974–92 in England and Wales. (Reproduced with permission of the OPCS (Crown copyright).)

and are thus potentially preventable. The increase is thought to be related to exposure to sunshine, particularly because of the rise in numbers of people holidaying and sunbathing abroad. The hypothesis that malignant melanoma is associated with sunbathing is supported by the fact that it is more common in the higher social classes (Fig. 18.10) and where Anglo-Saxon populations are resident in tropical regions such as Queensland (Australia) and parts of the USA. Young children who have been sunburnt have an increased risk of malignant melanoma later in life.

The Health of the Nation target is to halt the year-on-year increase in the incidence of skin cancer by 2005. Suggested strategies to achieve this goal include advice on the avoidance of sunlight (especially around midday in summer) and to encourage the use of barrier creams particularly for young children. A problem with a primary prevention programme to reduce the incidence of a cancer is that there is likely to be a long lag time between the initiation of the programme and changes in incidence or mortality.

MENTAL ILLNESS

The WHO has defined health as 'a state of complete physical, mental and

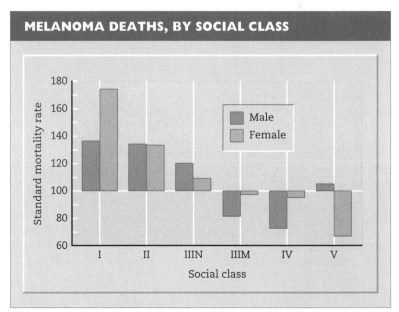

Fig. 18.10 Mortality from malignant melanoma in England by Registrar General's social class. N, non-manual; M, manual.

social well-being'. If this is the overall aim of the nation's health strategy then improving people's mental health must be included as a health target. Deaths attributed to mental illness are principally due to dementia and suicide. There are about 4000 suicides a year, the majority being in people under the age of 65 years. The incidence of suicide has risen in young men since 1972 and the rate in men far exceeds that in women (Fig. 18.11).

Mental illness is a major cause of morbidity and utilizes considerable health resources both from primary care and from the specialist mental health services. Around 1% of the population have a major functional psychosis at any one time and one in seven people see their general practitioner in any one year with neurosis (principally anxiety and depression). Prescriptions of antidepressants and anxiolytics are amongst the major items within the pharmaceutical budget. There is great scope to improve the efficiency and effectiveness of prescribing in this area. Currently, up to 75% of prescriptions for tricyclic antidepressants are at sub-therapeutic dosages. Thus, patients are exposed to their side effects without the likelihood of benefiting from the treatment. The Health of the Nation targets are as follows.

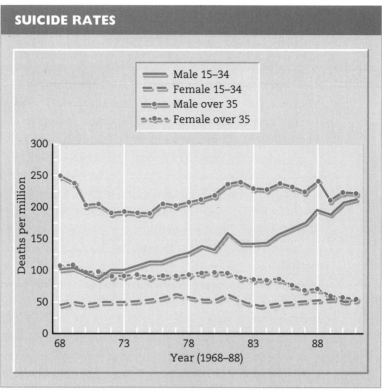

SUICIDE RATES

Legend:
- Male 15–34
- Female 15–34
- Male over 35
- Female over 35

Deaths per million

Year (1968–88)

Fig. 18.11 Suicides and undetermined deaths: all methods, in England and Wales. (Reproduced with permission of the OPCS (Crown copyright).)

TARGETS FOR MENTAL HEALTH

- To improve significantly the health and social functioning of mentally ill people
- To reduce the overall suicide rate by at least 15% by the year 2000
- To reduce the suicide rate of severely mentally ill people by at least 33% by the year 2000

The first priority in achieving the goals for mental health will be to improve the local and national collection of data and to introduce standardized assessment procedures. It is hoped that the development of comprehensive local services based on local joint planning and purchasing arrangements will ensure continuity of health and social care. Other suggested strategies include encouraging general practitioners to recognize and treat a higher proportion of depressed patients, to treat depression with antidepressants at full therapeutic dosages, to elicit an alcohol history from patients and, when appropriate, to take steps to reduce excessive drinking.

HIV/AIDS AND SEXUAL HEALTH

AIDS was first recognized in 1981 in the USA amongst young male homosexuals and it is now found in practically every country in the world. The WHO estimated in 1994 that between 13 and 14 million people were infected with HIV and that there were 6000 new cases every day. The majority of cases are in sub-Saharan Africa, where transmission is principally through heterosexual intercourse. Since reporting began in the UK in 1982, there have been 10 000 cases of AIDS reported, of whom 70% have died. Twenty-three thousand people were identified as HIV positive between 1985 (when a suitable test became available) and 1994 (Fig. 18.12).

Special characteristics of the epidemiology of AIDS have been crucial to identifying the groups most at risk and in providing strategies for the control of the disease.

In the UK, up to July 1995, 91% of patients with AIDS and 86% of those who were HIV positive (but did not all have AIDS) were men (Table 18.1). The spread of HIV amongst heterosexuals, however, is increasing. Immigrants from Africa (where the disease is predominantly transmitted

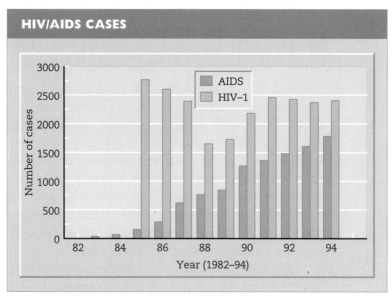

Fig. 18.12 Numbers of reports of HIV-1 and AIDS in the UK per year.

AIDS CASES AND DEATHS

How HIV infection was probably acquired	Male	Male (deaths)	Female	Female (deaths)
Sexual intercourse				
between men	8 101	5725	–	–
between men and women				
exposure to 'high-risk' partner(s)	40	20	117	68
exposure abroad	648	360	438	220
exposure in the UK	75	48	65	44
investigation incomplete	19	5	7	1
Injecting drug use	449	292	202	118
Blood factor treatment (e.g. for haemophilia)	493	424	6	5
Blood/tissue transfer (e.g. transfusion)	39	26	71	48
Mother to fetus	81	42	82	40
Other	100	76	18	9
Total	10 045	7018	1006	553

Table 18.1 AIDS cases and deaths by exposure category, UK, January 1982 to June 1995. (Source: *Comm. Dis. Rep.*; number 29.)

heterosexually) account for part of the increase in prevalence. Recently, the number of women infected has also been increasing due to sexual contact with men who are bisexual or intravenous drug users. It is likely that the trend of an increasing proportion of cases due to heterosexual contact will continue.

Most cases of AIDS in the UK until now have occurred in young to middle-aged homosexually active males. It was the marked number of cases amongst male homosexuals that led to the hypothesis that the most common form of transmission was through anal intercourse. The risk appears to be greater for the receptive partner. Studies in developing countries have shown that vaginal intercourse between heterosexuals is also an effective method of transmission of the virus. Again, it appears that the receptive (female) partner is more at risk. The presence of genital lesions due to other STDs may increase the chance of transmission.

HIV is also transmitted through blood and blood products. A large number of people were infected through blood transfusions carried out before the virus was recognized. A high proportion of haemophiliacs using untested factor VIII were infected. Intravenous drug users are also at increased risk through blood-borne transmission if they share needles or syringes.

Vertical transmission of HIV occurs from mother to fetus. It will become a more significant problem as the number of HIV-infected women increases. By April 1994, there were 643 HIV-infected women in the UK known to have delivered a baby. Currently, the transmission rate of HIV to the child is around 25%, but the avoidance of breast feeding, caesarean section and the use of zidovudine (an antiviral agent) during pregnancy seems to reduce this risk to less than 10%. These measures can only be considered when the HIV status of the mother is known antenatally. At present in the UK, information from anonymous testing indicates that four out of five mothers infected with HIV are unaware of their HIV status.

Because of the lack of effective treatment for HIV, control of the disease has rested principally on preventive strategies. The first priority was to ensure that all blood and blood products were safe. All donors are now screened for HIV and donors who are at high risk are asked not to offer themselves as donors. This has meant that the chances of contracting HIV through a blood transfusion, or through factor VIII for haemophiliacs, is now extremely small.

A key preventive strategy has been to change behaviour through education on safer sexual practices. At the same time, it is recognized that promotion of safe sex to stop the transmission of HIV will help control the spread of other STDs and may also lead to changes in contraceptive practice and family planning. Specific Health of the Nation targets for reducing the incidence of HIV infection were not set because of the uncertainty concerning the current baseline rates. However, targets for reduction in the frequency of drug misuse and gonorrhoea were intended as proxies for reducing the likelihood of HIV transmission.

Several specific strategies have been pursued in the UK to reduce HIV transmission. Safe sex has been promoted through advertising and education. Television has taken a lead in promoting the use of condoms especially to young people. Condoms have now become more widely available. The message of safe sex amongst homosexuals has been spread by means of community participation. Gay organizations have been active in trying to bring about changes in sexual behaviour. Health promotion campaigns have not been completely successful. There are still new cases of HIV being diagnosed in young homosexual men attending genito-urinary medicine clinics, indicating that the message concerning safe sex has not been universally heard, or if it has, it has not led to the required changes in behaviour.

Information and education is also used as an important strategy in trying to reduce the transmission of HIV amongst intravenous drug users. Government-sponsored needle exchange programmes and a more understanding approach to the identification and provision of health services for intravenous drug users has helped to control the spread of HIV in this group.

Screening for HIV is voluntary because of the consequences of the diagnosis to the individual. Considerable pretest counselling is required and the opportunity this offers to promote safe behaviour is also taken. Testing for HIV in genito-urinary medicine and antenatal clinics has been well accepted, but anonymous testing has shown that there are still many people who are infected but apparently unaware of their HIV status. The anonymous and voluntary screening that has occurred has given both useful epidemiological information and allowed more effective strategies to be planned.

AIDS and the workplace

When AIDS first appeared, uncertainty about the mode of transmission led to great anxiety amongst co-workers of infected individuals. Through education, much of this prejudice has gone. Changes have also occurred on sports fields where players with cuts are sent from the field for treatment.

It is probably in the area of health care that the greatest concern arises. Health workers are at risk from infected patients and occupational health practices have been tightened to protect staff and patients. Despite this, on rare occasions doctors and nurses have contracted the infection from patients and vice versa. The problem of the infected doctor or nurse and the risk they present to patients has been a major concern of public health physicians. There have been several well-publicized cases where surgeons, dentists or midwives have been found to be infected with HIV. In these circumstances, as with hepatitis B, it is mandatory for all the patients who have been exposed to risk to be identified and an assessment made of their risk. These patients then need to be contacted and offered a test for HIV to check they have not been infected. To date, more than 5000 patients in the UK have been contacted in these circumstances although none has been found to have been infected by the health worker involved. However, vigilance in the public interest must be maintained in such situations. The Health of the Nation targets related to sexual health, HIV and AIDS are as follows.

TARGETS FOR SEXUAL HEALTH

- To reduce the incidence of gonorrhoea among men and women aged 15–64 years by at least 20% by 1995
- To reduce the rate of conceptions among girls under 16 years by at least 50% by the year 2000
- To reduce the percentage of injecting drug misusers who report sharing injecting equipment in the previous 4 weeks by at least 50% by 1997 and by at least a further 50% by the year 2000

ACCIDENTS

In England, accidents result in about 9000 deaths per year and are the most common cause of death in people under 30 years of age. There is substantial variation in the numbers and in the types of accident with age and sex: the annual death rate in males aged 15–44 years is four times that of females in this age group.

The pattern of accidents varies enormously with environmental conditions and personal factors. For example, road accidents occur most frequently in the hours of darkness and in winter months, whereas drownings occur most frequently in the daytime in summer. Alcohol can be a significant factor in both. Nearly half of all deaths in children are the result of road traffic accidents, except in those under 5 years old in whom suffocation is the most common cause, followed by burns and scalds, falls and poisoning. There is a sharp peak in the incidence of road accident deaths in males in the 15–24 year age group, due in particular to motor cycle accidents (Fig. 18.13). This peak in road accidents is much less dramatic in females. In people over age 65 years, the frequency of accidental deaths increases, particularly as a result of falls in females (Fig. 18.14). Statistics such as these help to identify areas of risk in which there is a special need for preventive effort. The Health of the Nation targets are as follows.

TARGETS FOR ACCIDENTAL DEATH

- To reduce the death rate for accidents among children aged under 15 years by at least 33% by the year 2005
- To reduce the death rate for accidents among young people aged 15–24 years by at least 25% by the year 2005
- To reduce the death rate for accidents among people aged 65 years and over by at least 33% by the year 2005

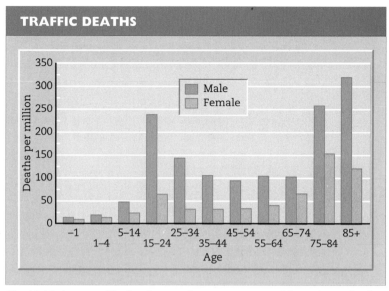

Fig. 18.13 Age-specific death rates from transport accidents in England, 1992. (Reproduced with permission of the OPCS (Crown copyright).)

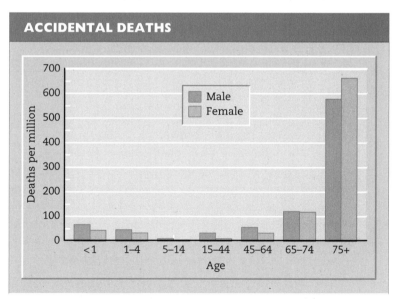

Fig. 18.14 Age-specific deaths from accidents in the home and in residential institutions in England, 1989. (Reproduced with permission of the OPCS (Crown copyright).)

The main strategies aimed at reducing accidental deaths in children and young adults include an emphasis on reducing the causal factors in road traffic deaths, i.e. drink-driving and excessive speed. People are also encouraged to wear their seat belts and to use safety seats for children.

Strategies to reduce poisonings include advice to keep medicines locked away from children. There are also suggestions within Health of the Nation that non-fatal sports injuries can be reduced by care in warming up and cooling down before and after sport.

For the over 65-year-olds, the messages are aimed principally at the prevention of falls by ensuring that landings and stairs are well lit, that people have their eyes checked regularly and that people who have had falls should have their homes checked for safety.

As well as the strategies suggested by the Health of the Nation, strategies aimed at improving the environment have proved effective in the past in reducing accidents.

ENVIRONMENTAL SAFETY

It is always preferable to create a safe environment than to rely on public education in safety. This is exemplified by action taken to improve road and home safety.

Road safety

This has been enhanced by improvements in road engineering, surfaces and furnishings, and better street lighting, combined with safety devices in the design of vehicles.

The 1967 Road Safety Act introduced regulations relating to drinking and driving. This was followed by a substantial fall in the number of serious accidents. Many countries have introduced laws making the wearing of seat belts compulsory for car drivers and passengers with the result that deaths and serious injuries from road accidents have been significantly reduced. Legislation already exists in the UK relating to worn tyres and other vehicle safety features; motor cyclists are required to wear crash helmets. Enforcement of these regulations, however, presents serious practical difficulties and their effectiveness can be limited.

Home safety

This has been improved by better design of domestic appliances (especially electrical and heating appliances), flame-proof children's clothing, and good housing design (especially the protection of stairs and balconies). Prevention also depends on maintaining the home and its contents in a good state of repair. Building regulations govern their safety in relation to fire hazards, ventilation, lighting and other matters. Regulations on the safety of domestic appliances also indirectly assist safety in the home.

It should be noted that environmental control, education and regulation are insufficient to eliminate accidents in all circumstances. For example, many motorcycle accidents are caused not by people using the motor cycle as a method of transport but as a way of testing nerve during late adolescence, almost amounting to a cult. Those who pursue these dangerous activities are well aware of the risks, and are prepared to accept the personal risks involved in exactly the same way as a mountaineer. Nor do they regard the risks imposed on others as a significant deterrent. The desire of adolescents to test the limits of their physical endurance is a natural phenomenon and hard to combat by any conventional preventive strategies.

PART 3

Health Services

CHAPTER 19

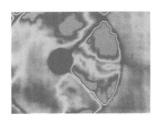

History and Principles

INTRODUCTION

Health services fall into two broad categories:
- personal health services;
- public or environmental health services.

Personal health services

These include the whole range of preventive, treatment and rehabilitative services provided for individuals. General practice is the main source of primary, domiciliary and ambulatory care. Specialist services tend to be concentrated in general hospitals managed by NHS acute trusts. Long-term care is organized through NHS community trusts and private and voluntary organizations. The preventive services are mainly provided through general practice but additional facilities are available in some areas through a variety of agencies.

Public health services

These are concerned with the control and prevention of disease in the community, advice on public policies for health promotion, assessment of the health care needs of the population and planning and evaluation of health services. The control and preventive function includes the monitoring of disease and the control of factors in the environment that may affect health such as the quality and safety of air, water, food, the control of occupational and industrial hazards and environmental pollution. In a complex industrial society, health may be affected by public policy in many fields that are not normally thought of as specifically 'health' services. For example, education, transport, housing, industrial, commercial and economic policies may all directly or indirectly influence the health and welfare of society. One of the functions of a public health service is to monitor these factors and to provide scientific evidence of their health implications. Public health doctors have traditionally been involved in the development and provision of health promotion strategies to try and alter these influences on health. More recently, they have been involved in health care needs assessment and in providing advice on the purchasing of health services as well as evaluating their effectiveness and efficiency. This role has been developed particularly at the local level within DHAs.

The history and evolution of both personal and public health services is described in this chapter. In Chapter 20, the present arrangements for the delivery of health services in England and Wales are described.

HISTORY OF PERSONAL HEALTH SERVICES

A characteristic of human societies is that they accept responsibility for the care of individuals who, through no fault of their own, are unable to care and provide for themselves. In general, these are the elderly, the poor and the disabled. The most basic expression of this obligation is care through the extended family, i.e. parents, siblings, children, uncles and aunts, together with others who identify with the family. The main unit of rural societies is the family. Here, families normally live close together and share the same type of work. In these circumstances the personal caring aspect of the family's life is absorbed into its normal activities. In modern industrial societies, families are more mobile, both geographically and socially, and work is normally a separate activity from day-to-day life. For this reason, even though the family may appreciate that it has a responsibility to those of its members who are unable to care for themselves, it is often not in a position to assist them. For example, different generations may live in different towns, or the daytime jobs of the main wage earners of a nuclear family may preclude them from devoting sufficient time to the care of an aged relative. Moreover, the role of women has changed from one of child bearer, child rearer and housekeeper to a partner in both domestic matters and wage earning. Therefore, services involving people other than the family have had to develop. Such involvement made it necessary to create a system of payment for care services and generated the need for professional carers. In modern societies, this is organized and funded by the State.

The process whereby personal health care evolved from being solely a family obligation to being a professional activity with state involvement in its financing and supervision was complex. It was influenced by the structure of societies, changes in the expectations of individuals and developments in medical science and technology.

In England, the earliest legislation for the public provision of services for the sick was the Act for the Relief of the Poor (1598) usually referred to as the Poor Law, which required parishes to appoint an 'overseer of the poor . . . to raise money by local taxation and to provide . . . the necessary relief for the lame, impotent, old, blind and other such being poor and not able to work.' This legislation implicitly recognized the relationship between disablement and poverty and it restricted help to those who had no other source of support. In effect, it was a last-resort provision. It was not fully repealed until the passage of the NHS Act in 1946.

Early arrangements for the care of the sick were rudimentary. They were provided with shelter, food and basic care. The roles of the doctors and of medicine were limited principally to the care of the wealthy, except through the major charitable hospitals. During the twentieth century there has been dramatic progress in the development of medical skills and of medical technology. These have affected the shape of medical services in many ways. The new special skills and technologies had to be concentrated in institutions (hospitals) in order that they could develop. This brought about a change in the nature of the hospital from an institution concerned with the general care of the poor to one that was clearly medically orientated. Many people who in previous generations had been looked after at home, turned to hospitals for investigation, care and treatment. Consequently, the social mix of hospital patients changed and they ceased to be the last refuge of the neglected, the destitute and those whose families had dispersed. This changed the standards and nature of care offered within the hospitals.

THE MEDICAL PROFESSION

DOCTORS

Until the middle of the nineteenth century there were three types of medical practitioners in the UK:
- Physicians
- Surgeons
- Apothecaries

Nearly all of these worked almost entirely outside hospitals

Physicians

These were university graduates (mainly from Oxford and Cambridge) who had then qualified for a diploma of the Royal College of Physicians (founded in 1518). Their background was upper class and their practice was mainly among the upper and merchant classes. They attended the voluntary hospitals on a charitable basis.

Surgeons

These qualified with a diploma from the Royal College of Surgeons (founded in 1800). They frequently worked under the supervision of the physicians.

Apothecaries

The third group, who co-existed with the physicians and surgeons, were the apothecaries. Strictly, they were apprentice-trained tradesmen whose qualification was in making medicines rather than in diagnosis and prescribing. Although they did act as doctors, they were breaking the law in pursuing such activities. They extended their activities during the plague in the seventeenth century, when most physicians left London together with other members of the upper classes. Then, by default, the apothecaries adopted a new role. By the beginning of the nineteenth century, the apothecaries were well established as doctors to all but the upper classes. They were not, however, appointed to the honorary staff of the voluntary hospitals.

THE GMC

In 1853, physicians, surgeons and apothecaries were placed on a common register maintained by the GMC which was charged by law with control over training and qualifications. The GMC still regulates the profession and is responsible for setting standards of education, the registration of medical practitioners and dealing with complaints about a doctor's fitness to practice. Only graduates who have undergone the prescribed training and passed the appropriate exams can be registered. Members of the public who are dissatisfied with the conduct or performance of any registered medical practitioner may complain to the GMC who will then investigate the complaint and may take action against the doctor which can include the removal of the doctor from the register.

HOSPITALS

Voluntary hospitals

A few hospitals were established in England by religious orders during the Middle Ages. These include St Bartholomew's and St Thomas's Hospitals in London. They were founded as practical demonstrations of Christian charity to provide care for the destitute. By 1700, there were fewer than 12 such hospitals in the whole country, most of which were in London. The period during which the greatest number of hospitals were built was in the late eighteenth and nineteenth centuries.

The voluntary hospitals were supported at first by church funds, charitable contributions and endowments. They were founded principally as places of asylum and rest for the physically sick and chronically disabled. They were staffed by unpaid doctors (consultants) and, in the teaching hospitals, by doctors in training. Their location was determined in part by local need and in part by the availability of 'private practice' for the honorary staff, which was their only source of income. Outside the main teaching centres, there were other types of voluntary hospital, including cottage hospitals, funded locally and staffed by local general practitioners on a part-time basis.

The advent of more sophisticated medical treatments and diagnostic techniques, developed largely in the London teaching hospitals, made the voluntary hospitals become more selective in their admissions. They tended to admit patients whose stay was likely to be short and to avoid admitting the chronically sick. Such patients were either admitted to or transferred to municipal hospitals.

By the end of the nineteenth century, the patients of the major voluntary hospitals were no longer limited to the destitute. Because of the increasing costs of providing a service, they had to introduce a system of payment for those who could afford to pay. The charitable funds were used for those who could not. Most hospitals employed 'lady almoners' whose job it was to establish who should be subsidized and to what extent. Despite the introduction of a semi fee-paying system, the costs of maintaining these hospitals rose faster than their incomes and they became increasingly financially embarrassed.

At the outbreak of the Second World War the Government set up the Emergency Medical Service in order to meet the large number of military and civilian casualties that were expected. This guaranteed money to the voluntary hospitals to meet the predicted need. After the war, lack of a secure income made a return to their former independent status impossible. Most of them were incorporated into the NHS in 1948.

Municipal hospitals

The Elizabethan Poor Law enabled parishes to attach infirmary wards to workhouses. Parishes were small population units and in order to produce a viable system, groups of parishes combined to administer the Poor Law legislation. These groups were called parish unions. Boards of guardians appointed by the unions were responsible for the day-to-day administration of the institutions.

The Poor Law infirmaries were for the destitute sick and were quite unlike hospitals as we know them today. At first, they did not have any medical staff: nursing care was provided by the non-sick inmates of the workhouse. Over the years, the infirmaries improved, although there was considerable variation in standards. A feature of much of the Poor Law legislation and the legislation governing matters of public health was that, although it gave local authorities discretionary powers to improve the standards and scope of care, it did not place a duty on them to do so. In this lies one of the reasons for the present maldistribution of health care resources in the UK. The Poor Law infirmaries were made over to local government authorities in 1929. They then became municipal hospitals. From then until the outbreak of the Second World War a concerted effort was made to improve standards and staffing. In 1939, the municipal hospitals were grouped with the voluntary hospitals in regions as part of the Emergency Medical Service.

Other hospitals

There were two other types of public hospitals during the first half of the twentieth century; fever hospitals and lunatic asylums.

The fever hospitals were established to protect the public from infection. Only later were they able to offer treatment. Among them were large numbers of tuberculosis sanitoria. These were built between the two world wars and are testaments to the high prevalence of that disease and to increasing faith in its treatment.

The lunatic asylums had a chequered history. Until 1890, the mentally disturbed were cared for in private mad houses (some with appalling reputations) or in prison or in workhouses (not the workhouse infirmary which was established for the physically sick).

The Lunacy Act of 1890 placed a duty on county authorities to provide asylums for those of unsound mind. The London County Council built many such hospitals including nine, with accommodation for several thousand patients, around Epsom in Surrey. The distance from London did not deter the planners as they took it for granted that once patients were admitted there was little chance that they would ever be discharged.

DOMICILIARY HEALTH SERVICES

National Health Insurance Act

The Poor Law Commission (1909) demonstrated that a lack of early medical advice often resulted in prolonged sickness and consequent poverty. Its findings led to the introduction of the National Health Insurance Act in 1911. The important provisions of this Act were as follows.

THE NATIONAL HEALTH INSURANCE ACT (1911)

- Free medical treatment from a general practitioner who the insured person was free to choose (provided the doctor had agreed to participate in the scheme)
- Doctors who participated in the scheme were paid on a capitation basis, i.e. so much per year per person registered. This was advantageous to the general practitioner as it guaranteed him a regular income for the first time
- Weekly payments to insured persons while sick to enable them to maintain minimal living standards

The scheme was restricted to working men whose income was below a specified minimum amount. It did not include retired persons, the wives of working men or their children. The scheme was administered by approved Friendly Societies. In subsequent years, the National Insurance scheme was extended and, by 1945, the majority of the population was covered.

General practice

Specialities developed in the hospitals because of the facilities offered there, while the doctors who worked mainly in the community became known as general practitioners. The majority of the population paid their general practitioner a fee for consultation. In the growing conurbations, the fact that people could be seen free of charge in the out-patient departments of the voluntary hospitals caused some resentment among general practitioners. In order to overcome this, a system was developed whereby patients would only be seen in out-patients if referred by their regular doctor.

Domiciliary nursing

At the beginning of the nineteenth century there were few trained nurses. The need for home nursing was appreciated by the middle of the century and in 1887 the Queen's Institute of District Nursing was established. The Institute set and maintained standards of practice and coordinated local voluntary committees.

MOTHERS AND INFANTS

The extremely high maternal and infant mortality in the nineteenth century led social reformers to look for ways of preventing this waste of life. Important landmarks were as follows.

• Foundation of the Manchester and Salford Sanitary Association, 1862. This organization employed women to give instruction and guidance to mothers on child rearing. The scheme eventually developed into what is now known as health visiting.

• The Midwives Act, 1902. This prohibited untrained women from practising midwifery.

• The Maternity and Child Welfare Act, 1918. This obliged local authorities to provide a medical service for expectant mothers, nursing mothers and children under 5 years of age.

• The Midwives Act, 1936. This made local authorities responsible for ensuring that there were sufficient midwives to meet the population's need.

THE NHS ACT (1946)

This Act had three major effects:
- It ensured everyone had free access to a general practitioner
- It brought the municipal and voluntary hospitals under the control of the (then) Ministry of Health
- It gave added responsibility to the Medical Officer of Health and local authorities in the running of community services

THE PRESENT TASKS OF PERSONAL MEDICAL SERVICES

The changes in medical practice during the past 50 years have been revolutionary. Today, access to complex technology, skilled personnel and powerful therapies is taken for granted. Some illnesses that were inaccessible to medical intervention a generation ago, can be treated by methods that are now commonplace. In all branches of medicine, however, there remains a need for the traditional role of the doctor, that of an informed professional carer. In some cases, medicine still has little to offer other than palliation and understanding; in others, once the correct diagnosis has been made the doctor's role is simply one of supervising long-term management.

Fortunately, most of the population is fit and well for most of the time; they only require access to medicine when they become sick. Broadly, the sick can be divided into those who require access to the modern technology of medicine both for the investigation and treatment of their illnesses and those for whom such facilities are less important than access to carers who have a thorough understanding of them as people and the effects the illness is having upon them. A modern health service must provide facilities, sensitive to individual need, that are accessible to everyone who becomes sick and appropriate caring services for the chronic sick and disabled.

Primary care

Primary care services are required for the whole population and for most people they are the first contact with the organized health services. They should enable individuals who become ill, or think they have a medical problem, to obtain advice, treatment or sometimes referral to a specialist service. Primary care services are provided in general practice, occupational health services, accident and emergency departments, first aid rooms and many other places. The precise location of primary care facilities varies from country to country: in most societies there are many alternative sources of such care.

Secondary care

Secondary care is concerned with the provision of specialist services which are usually provided within hospitals. Medical care that is dependent upon expensive diagnostic and treatment technology is concentrated in hospitals in order to maximize the use of costly equipment and skilled personnel. The task of specialist services is to diagnose, to initiate treatment and, when the equipment to treat is only available at the hospital, to complete the course of treatment.

Tertiary care

Increasingly, with further sophistication of medical technology a third or tertiary level of care has evolved. This provides specialty services on a regional or sometimes national basis and usually only accepts referrals from a consultant. Services that are considered tertiary specialties include neonatal intensive care, cardiac surgery, neurosurgery, renal services and oncology. These are high-cost services that need to be used efficiently and with discimination.

Continuing care

Another type of care is required for the long-term sick and those who do not require the facilities of a high-technology hospital. Ideally, this should be provided as close to the residence of the patient as possible. Sometimes it is feasible to provide it at home. Much of the work of general practice falls into this category and most of this type of care is in fact provided by general practitioners. About 80% of the consultations (whether in the surgery or at the patient's home) with general practitioners are generated by about 20% of the population. A large proportion of that 20% are the chronic sick who depend entirely on the general practitioner and his or her primary care team for their medical care. A number of community trusts have been set up to provide continuing care in the community in conjunction with general practitioners. There are other sources of continuing care. These include psychiatric units, institutions for the care of people with learning disabilities, geriatric units, hospices for the dying, homes for the young chronic sick and centres for those disabled by serious permanent injury or disease. In the past, the decision to provide long-term care in a specialist institution rather than in the patient's own home was affected more by the social circumstances and the availability of the family and friends to provide basic support than by the patient's medical condition. Today, cost is also a consideration and if people can be supported cost effectively in the community by professional carers then this option is increasingly being pursued.

Preventive medicine

Personal health care services must include easy access to preventive medicine activities (immunization, screening, health education, etc.). This is provided in a variety of ways including mother and child clinics, school clinics, well-women clinics, occupational health centres and general practice. In the absence of such resources, many avoidable illnesses will occur to the disadvantage of the individuals and society as a whole.

The role of the general practitioner is very broad but few of the activities are exclusive to him or her. The most expensive areas in the provision of medical care are the acute hospitals. It is hard for any society to achieve an ideal balance in its provision of services and there will always be a need to modify provision in the light of the circumstances of each community. In general, rich countries can afford the luxury of expensive technology but poorer and developing countries need to concentrate their sparse resources on personal preventive services, primary care and secondary care that is not dependent on expensive medical technology.

PUBLIC HEALTH SERVICES

Until the early nineteenth century, there was little public demand for state intervention in matters of health and welfare. During the 1820s and 1830s the so-called 'sanitary reform movement' began to gain momentum. It was particularly promoted by the lawyer and philosopher Jeremy Bentham. Bentham led the push for reform and encouraged the notion that the State should bear some responsibility for the health of its people. His ideas were carried on by his followers of whom the most notable was Edwin Chadwick. Chadwick produced a 'Report on the Sanitary Condition of the Labouring Population of Great Britain' in 1842 which highlighted the economic costs of an unhealthy workforce. This approach gained some support in Parliament and led to the Nuisances Removal Act (1846) which gave local authorities the power to clean up the towns though this was not a requirement on the authority. In 1847, Liverpool appointed the country's first Medical Officer of Health, Dr W.H. Duncan. The next year, the first Public Health Act (1848) was passed in the wake of a disastrous outbreak of cholera. This Act which encouraged, but did not compel, local authorities to employ Medical Officers of Health also appointed the first national authority with a responsibility for health in England – the General Board of Health. Opposition led to the disbanding of the Board in 1854. Despite its demise, further public health legislation continued to be passed including the 1871 Act (during a major smallpox epidemic), and the Public Health Act (1875) which obliged local authorities to improve provisions for the disposal of sewage, to provide pure water supplies and street cleaning, to improve housing standards, and many other aspects of urban life. The authorities were also then obliged to appoint Medical Officers of Health to advise them on matters relating to the health of the community. Interestingly, occupational health services were not included in this legislation and remain outside the NHS to the present day.

In the 1880s the discovery of many agents of infectious diseases began and public health entered the so-called 'Germ Theory Era' in which microbes were recognized as the causes of many of the most significant diseases of the time. This led to a more scientific approach to the control of infectious diseases. The value of the sanitary reforms then became evident, but the importance of isolation and quarantine, as well as personal and communal hygiene measures, in preventing the transmission of infectious diseases was recognized. The provision of vaccination against smallpox had been a state responsibility since the Vaccination Act (1853) but vaccination against other infectious diseases made little impact until the mid twentieth century.

When local authorities were established in their modern form in the nineteenth century, one of their principal roles was to administer environmental health services. Over the years, they have acquired a range of other functions, but their environmental health departments, staffed by Environmental Health Officers, continue to be the principal local agencies responsible for monitoring and enforcing many aspects of environmental standards, for example food, water supplies and sewage disposal, air quality, housing, and working conditions other than in factories (which are the responsibility of the Health and Safety Executive). They also carry statutory responsibility for the investigation and control of communicable disease in the community, obtaining medical advice for this and other purposes from doctors (consultants in public health medicine) employed by the corresponding DHAs.

The Ministry of Health was created in 1919 to exert more effective control over local bodies in the field of public health. The last important Public Health Act before the National Health Service Act was passed in 1936. It codified and simplified practice relating to environmental and personal hygiene. Thus, by 1946, public environmental health practice and its administration had evolved a structure close to its modern pattern but it remained separate from provision of the treatment of the sick.

Recently, the term 'The New Public Health' has come into use (see Chapter 12). Two books were published in the mid 1970s: The Medical Nemesis by I. Illich and The Role of Medicine—Dream, Mirage or Nemesis by T. McKeown which challenged the importance of high-technology medicine in improving the population's health status and promoted the view that improvements in the nutrition, housing and wealth of the people were the most significant factors in improving life expectancy and reducing morbidity over the last century. The economic recession caused by the oil crisis of the early 1970s led to a curtailing of spending on health care. This and the escalating costs of modern medicine encouraged a search for alternative ways to improve the peoples' health. The WHO began to expound the concepts of 'Health for All' based on preventive strategies and universal access to basic health services. A WHO meeting held in Southern Russia in 1978 formulated the Alma Ata Declaration on Primary Care. This Declaration proposed a number of strategies for improving health, and emphasized that primary care should be the main focus of national health services in all countries.

It was in the context of financial stringency and growing appreciation of the influences of environmental and economic and social factors on health that the UK Government commissioned a study led by Sir Douglas Black to examine inequalities in health. The Black Report entitled 'Social Inequality and Health' was published in 1980 and despite initial political resistance became a major influence on public health doctors' thinking about ways to improve health. At the same time, the WHO officially adopted 'Health for All by the Year 2000' as policy: this included a commitment to the idea of equity in health (both within and between countries), a commitment to community consultation and a greater emphasis on prevention and health promotion as strategies to improve health. The 'Health for All' strategy was adopted by the European Region of WHO who modified and developed appropriate health targets for Europe. These targets included proposed changes to the structure and process of health care as well as detailing targets on specific health outcomes. In the early 1980s, the city of Toronto took the WHO concepts of 'Health for All' and, using community consultation, came up with a plan for a 'Healthy City'. This involved collaboration between the health service agencies and the city authorities; it generated a number of projects which aimed to improve the city environment and people's health. The idea of Healthy Cities was quickly adopted by the European Region of the WHO and trials of the strategy of intersectoral collaboration were instigated in a number of European cities. In the UK, Liverpool became one of the first European cities to embrace this concept and soon over 120 cities world-wide were involved in implementing the Healthy City strategy.

In the UK, in pursuit of the 'Health for All' strategy, the DoH in 1991 published a document entitled 'The Health of the Nation' which set out a number of goals for improving public health. This again emphasized a commitment to the pursuit of health, as well as the provision of health care. The strategy involves prioritizing objectives, setting targets and monitoring and reviewing progress. The current targets are outlined in Chapter 18.

PUBLIC HEALTH DOCTORS

In 1974, the Medical Officers of Health and their personal health service responsibilities were brought into the NHS. At the same time, they, together with doctors working in medical administration and in relevant university departments, joined forces to form the new specialty of 'community medicine'. An erosion of the standards in some areas of traditional public health became apparent in the early 1980s, illustrated by a number of serious outbreaks of infectious diseases. This led the Government to set up an enquiry into the public health function. The subsequent report, 'Public Health in England' (Acheson, 1988), recommended a return to the old title of Public Health Medicine and doctors specializing in this field are now called public health physicians. The report redefined their role as outlined on page 253.

ROLE OF PUBLIC HEALTH PHYSICIANS (1988)

- To enquire into all matters which affect the health of communities or population groups
- To measure health care needs
- To plan, administer and evaluate services, with particular reference to the prevention of disease
- To promote health in the community
- To provide relevant advice to health authorities, central Government and other bodies

In addition, it was recommended that there should be a cadre of public health physicians with special training in communicable disease control.

Today, public health physicians have four major areas of responsibility.

- To advise on the purchase of health services. These doctors usually work for health authorities and are responsible for assessing the health care needs of populations, advising on the purchasing of appropriate services and the evaluation of their effectiveness and efficiency. Many of these doctors develop areas of special expertise such as the provision of acute or special needs services, or primary care. At the same time, an understanding of the demographic and social structure of populations and the dynamics of change is extremely important.
- The control of communicable diseases. This is the responsibility of public health physicians with special training in the epidemiology of infection, microbiology and clinical infectious diseases. These specialists work either in health authorities or in the national CDSCs. They are responsible for surveillance of communicable diseases, investigation of outbreaks and the instigation of control and preventive measures.
- Research in epidemiology and public health. Research in public health is an expanding area involving a multidisciplinary approach which incorporates statistics, social sciences, health economics and information technology. Specialist areas of research are also developing such as health services research, pharmaco-epidemiology and global health, as well as in the more traditional areas concerned with study of the causes and prevention of disease. Most of this work is undertaken in academic departments.
- The design, management and evaluation of health promotion activities. Health promotion is often initiated at either a national or regional level, and public health physicians with a special interest are usually involved in the identification of issues, the design of appropriate programmes and in arranging their evaluation.

Public health physicians are often in the forefront of changes in health services and their roles and responsibilities can change rapidly. For example, some NHS trusts are now seeking to employ public health physicians as medical directors to advise them in their role as service providers. In future, consortia of general practice fundholders may also employ public health physicians' skills to help develop more appropriate and efficient ways of providing services. Whatever the future, it seems certain that a population perspective of health and the expertise of those trained in the relevant specialties will always be essential in a public health service.

CHAPTER 20

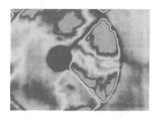

The National Health Service

ORIGINS

The important report by Sir William Beveridge on social and allied services, published in 1942, was the culmination of many years of pressure for social reform. It recommended that the State should finance and provide a comprehensive social security system and that it should be underpinned by a comprehensive national health service. It specifically proposed that a national health service should provide the facilities which would: '... ensure that for every citizen there is available whatever medical treatment he requires in whatever form he requires it, domiciliary or institutional, general, specialist or consultant, and will ensure also the provision of dental, ophthalmic and surgical appliances, nursing and midwifery, and rehabilitation after accidents'.

Apart from humanitarian considerations, which were the principal motivations for the proposals, Beveridge made the apparently logical assertion that such a health service would reduce the costs of social security payments by decreasing the amount of illness in the population. It was thought that this would increase the general appeal of the proposals. When estimating the possible costs of a health service, Beveridge and his colleagues made a further, and, as it turned out, disastrously naive assumption. They assumed that, as the health of the population improved because of the abolition of poverty, better preventive medicine and the elimination of the long-standing pool of untreated chronic illness, the cost of the proposed National Health Service would fall. They failed to anticipate the possibility of changes in the expectations of the public, the consequences of an ageing population and increases in the costs of medical technology.

The wartime coalition government accepted Beveridge's proposals for comprehensive national social security and health care systems but was unable to implement them immediately. It charged the Minister of Health for England and Wales, and the Secretary of State for Scotland with the responsibility of initiating consultations with representatives of the medical profession, the voluntary hospitals and the local authorities. Discussions began early in 1943 and on 8 February 1944 a White Paper on 'The National Health Service' (Cmd. 6502) was published. Its stated objective was: '. . . to show what is meant by a comprehensive service and how it fits with what has been done in the past, or is being done in the present, and so help people to look at the matter for themselves'. The publication of the White Paper served to crystallize ideas and to stimulate criticism. By the end of 1944 the Minister of Health submitted the suggestions that he had received from all interested parties to the Government. Basically, the proposals involved the Government taking financial and other responsibilities for the municipal, voluntary and other hospitals, for the general practitioner services as set up under the 1911 Act, and for municipal public health services and other aspects of personal and preventive medical services. Access to all services was to be without direct charges at the time of use for all residents of the country. In essence, the availability of the then existing services was to be extended, but their basic philosophy and administration changed little. On 19 March 1946, a Bill providing for the establishment of a comprehensive health service was presented to Parliament. Royal Assent was given to the National Health Service Act on 6 November 1946 and the Service was launched in July 1948.

THE NATIONAL HEALTH SERVICE, 1948

The administration of the original health service was divided into:
• Hospital services
• General practitioner services
• Local authority services

HOSPITAL SERVICES

Fourteen regional hospital boards were established within which there were 290 hospital groups each administered by a hospital management committee. The teaching hospitals (both undergraduate and postgraduate) were autonomous from the regional hospital boards. Each had their own board of governors which worked in close cooperation with the governing body of the associated university institution.

GENERAL PRACTITIONER SERVICES

The administration of general medical services was the responsibility of 134 executive councils. They administered:
• general medical services (family doctors);
• general dental services;
• pharmaceutical services;
• ophthalmic services.

All of the above services were, and still are, provided on an independent contractual basis. This means that the doctors, dentists, opticians, ophthalmic medical practitioners and pharmacists are not employed by the NHS; they are paid by the NHS for the services they provide. The executive councils had limited disciplinary and planning functions, their main role was that of a paying agency. Technically, general practitioners and other independent contractors were directly accountable to the Minister. In effect, the contractual position of this group of practitioners was little different to that under the 1911 legislation except that the services were now available free to all citizens.

LOCAL AUTHORITY SERVICES

The local government authorities were responsible for the care and aftercare of patients in the community and with the prevention of disease. Specifically they were responsible for:
• antenatal care;
• midwifery;
• infant and child welfare;
• district (domiciliary) nursing;
• health visiting;
• school health services;
• immunization;
• ambulance services;
• environmental health and a number of other functions relating to the control of infectious disease.

EARLY PROBLEMS

In its early years, the NHS experienced many difficulties and shortcomings. The most significant of these were as follows.

• There had been a gross underestimation of the cost of the service. The estimated first year cost of the NHS was £179 million. It actually cost £400 million.

• The NHS inherited many old and small hospitals, which had been built under the Poor Law provisions. After the Second World War, the Government's first priority was to build houses rather than hospitals. As a result there was almost no new hospital building for the first 20 years of the existence of the NHS.

• The division of administration of the service between three bodies (hospitals, general practitioners and public health) resulted in lack of coordination and cooperation. For example, many hospitals served several different local authority areas; and all three divisions of the service were involved in maternity services.

The NHS had failed to correct the long-standing inequalities in service provision between different parts of the country and between different types of service. The most neglected services were the care of the aged, the mentally ill, and people with learning disabilities together with services for the chronic sick and disabled. The northern regions of the country were poorly provided with hospitals but the areas in and around London had an historical, relatively overgenerous provision. The continued geographical maldistribution of facilities was at least partly due to the fact that there was inadequate capital investment in new hospitals in under-provided regions.

CHANGES IN THE 1970S AND 1980S

The original tripartite structure of the NHS was seen as a hindrance to the achievement of an integrated and balanced service throughout the country. As a result of a series of enquiries and reports by advisory groups in the 1960s, a major reorganization of the NHS occurred in 1974. The most important aspects of that reorganization were that the country was divided into a number of regional health authorities (RHAs) within each of which there was a number of area health authorities (AHAs) each of which was in turn subdivided into districts (DHAs). The authorities were responsible for the provision of all services other than the independent contractor services within their geographical boundaries. They thus took over many of the responsibilities that had been left with the local authorities in 1948. Where possible, the geographical boundaries of the health authorities were aligned with those of the local government authorities. The independent contractors (general medical practice, general dental practice, pharmaceutical service, ophthalmic services, etc.) became the responsibility of family practitioner committees. The RHAs had a mainly strategic planning and financial control role, the AHAs planned and managed some of the specialist services whilst the DHAs were responsible for the day-to-day management. In 1975, the Resource Allocation Working Party (RAWP) was appointed to address some of the inconsistencies of funding between regions but not to advise on the total level of funding for the service. Prior to the 1974 reorganization, expenditure per person in some regions was only 55% of that of the richest region. RAWP's main objective was to ensure that 'there would eventually be equal opportunity of access to health care for people at equal risk'. RAWP did not take into account general practitioner services, local authority services or those provided by the private sector. Since RAWP there has been substantial redirection of resources to certain less well provided areas.

In 1982, the AHAs were abolished. Some of their responsibilities were transferred to the RHAs and others to the DHAs.

In the 1980s, there was a renaissance of the philosophy that optimum efficiency within an organization was best obtained by exposing the organization to market forces. At the same time, there was a move away from the principle of state ownership. However, the State retained responsibility for politically sensitive areas including health and education whilst at the same time introducing the principles of the market place into these services. In the late 1980s, the financial restrictions placed on institutions by health authorities led some hospitals to seek an alternative funding structure. The idea of independent hospital trusts was born. A bill was passed to allow the creation of NHS trusts which would be funded directly from the DoH. The move to trust status was to be voluntary and initially most hospitals chose to remain as directly managed units of DHAs. Another key reform enabled general practitioners to hold funds on behalf of their patients including budgets for medicines and some secondary services such as non-urgent surgical and medical services, for example orthopaedics, dermatology etc. These general practitioners could then choose whether to use their funds to purchase services from the local hospital, from a trust or from the private sector. Choices could be made on the basis of quality and availability of service or on price or a combination of the two. There was an expectation that the introduction of competition into the NHS would control costs and improve quality through the pressure of an artificial market. At the same time, the contract between general practitioners and hospitals became more explicit.

THE PRESENT MANAGEMENT ARRANGEMENTS

The principles that govern the management of the service are that the health authorities have responsibility for purchasing health services for the population of their geographical areas and that, within general strategies and financial limits they have considerable autonomy to allow them to respond to local needs. The general strategies and financial allocations are decided by the Government and the NHS Management Board. These are transmitted via the RHAs to be implemented by the DHAs (Fig. 20.1).

The Secretary of State for Health is responsible to Parliament for the NHS and as a member of the Cabinet is able to bring the needs of the Service to the attention of the Government and to argue the case for necessary funds. The Secretary of State is also responsible for the enactment of government policy on health matters accounting to Parliament for the expenditure of the Service and for its performance. The Secretary of State is responsible to Parliament for:

- promoting and protecting the health of the nation;
- providing a national health service in England;

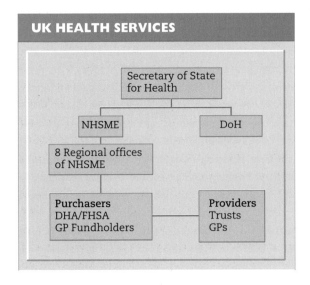

Fig. 20.1 Organization of health services in the UK, 1996.

• social care including oversight of personal social services provided by local authorities in England.

The DoH in England provides administrative support to the Secretary of State and the departmental ministers. Its main functions are to assist them by supplying the information they need regarding the working of the service, to advise them on the choices available when making policy decisions and the possible consequences of the available options, to transmit policy decisions to the regions, and to monitor progress in their achievement. Similar responsibilities are exercised by the Secretaries of State for Scotland, Wales and Northern Ireland, supported by counterpart administrative arrangements.

NHS MANAGEMENT EXECUTIVE

The NHS Executive is concerned with:
• Regional liaison matters
• NHS manpower
• NHS finance
• NHS support services (building design, maintenance, equipment, etc.)

REGIONAL HEALTH AUTHORITIES

In 1994, the 14 RHAs in England were reduced to eight which now function as regional offices of the NHS Management Executive. These offices distribute funds to the purchasing agencies which are the DHAs and family health service authorities (FHSAs). In many districts, these two authorities have combined to form single district commissioning agencies.

In order to purchase services on behalf of their communities effectively, purchasing agencies must understand the health needs of their communities. Consequently they have developed demographic profiles, and local information on mortality and morbidity rates. In addition, community health councils, which represent various interests in the corresponding local communities, can offer advice on local health needs. DHAs sometimes undertake or commission studies to help their decision making on particular health problems.

Purchasers are not restricted to purchasing services from their local providers. In theory they can purchase services from whomsoever they wish. Some services may be provided by both general practitioners and specialists, for example many chronic conditions such as diabetes, care of the elderly or care for people with learning disabilities can be managed either by primary care teams or from hospital-based clinics. Decisions on where to purchase care, and the balance between types of services can vary according to current priorities, perceived quality of care, overall outcomes and cost.

DISTRICT HEALTH AUTHORITIES

The District General Manager (or Chief Executive of a commissioning agency) is responsible to the authority for the performance of the service and advises on planning and strategic matters. He or she also liaises closely with the permanent staff of the regional office of the management executive in order to advise them of the local situation and be appraised of their medium and long-term plans. He or she is supported by district directors of public health, finance, planning, personnel, information and information technology. Within each of the districts there is a series of professional advisory committees. District General Managers are not obliged to consult the advisory committees before making a management decision nor do they have to accept any of the advice that they are given.

FAMILY HEALTH SERVICE AUTHORITIES

The FHSAs are responsible for the supervision of services provided for the NHS by independent practitioners under contract with them. These are general medical practitioners, general dental practitioners, ophthalmic and dispensing opticians and pharmaceutical contractors. While none of these is employed by the NHS, each contracts with the NHS through the FHSA to provide specified services. The geographical areas covered by the FHSA hitherto often included more than one DHA, but many DHAs and FHSAs have combined to provide a unified purchasing agency and in future this is likely to be the norm. This should facilitate coordination of developments such as health centres.

Each FHSA currently has 30 members who are appointed to include representatives of the DHAs, the relevant local authorities, the local medical committee, the local dental committee, the local pharmaceutical committee, ophthalmic opticians and dispensing opticians. There is also a number of 'lay' members. The FHSA elects its own chairman and has a full-time manager with a large clerical staff.

Local medical committees are comprised of general practitioners elected by their colleagues. Their role is to advise the FHSA. Local dental and pharmaceutical committees have corresponding functions.

COMMUNITY HEALTH COUNCILS

These were set up by the former RHAs to represent the interests of the public in health service matters. Their membership comprises representatives of local voluntary organizations concerned with health, and members of the local authority. Although they are statutory bodies, they have no executive role. They have certain rights of access to health service premises and to information relevant to their role. They also have the right to comment on the DHA's plans and to make alternative proposals which the DHA is obliged to consider.

NHS TRUSTS

Most specialist services are provided by NHS trusts which, although part of the NHS and accountable to their regional office, have considerable authority within broad guidelines. Each trust has a board of trustees and a chief executive officer. There are three main types of trusts.

• Acute care trusts. These manage large district hospitals and sometimes regional or tertiary services.

• Mental health trusts. These provide mental health services, including psychiatric in-patient units, community mental health services and in some cases forensic services. In some districts, mental health services are run by acute trusts or community trusts.

• Community trusts. These provide community services such as district nursing and health visiting. In addition, some community trusts provide minor accident centres, community physiotherapy, immunization clinics, etc. In some areas, these services are provided through acute care trusts.

Where general practitioners are fundholders, they can, by judicious use of their purchasing power, directly influence the range and quality of services provided by trusts. In some instances, the benefits of these changes are available only to patients from fundholding practices, leading to accusations that a two-tier health service is developing. Some general practitioners have formed large purchasing consortia which have the advantage of enhancing their purchasing power whilst reducing the costs of administration. These are called multifunds. They may include as many as 100 general practitioners.

LOCAL AUTHORITIES

Local authorities have purchasing powers similar to those of the health authorities, particularly in respect of services for the elderly, some mental health services and services for those with learning disabilities.

CARE OF THE ELDERLY

The local authority has the primary responsibility for ensuring that the necessary range of care for the elderly–from sheltered accommodation through to rest home care – is provided. Payment for this accommodation is means tested. Thus, where elderly people are ready for discharge from hospital care but are unable to support themselves, they can either be returned home supported by community health workers or be accommodated in a rest home. If they are moved to accommodation provided through social services, they are obliged to pay all or part of the costs whilst they have the resources to do so.

Other social services support may include the alteration of the home to make it more suitable for home care. The need for such alterations is assessed by the occupational therapist who in England is usually employed by the local authority. In addition, local authorities employ social workers who liaise between the health agencies and the Social Services Department.

MENTAL ILLNESS

The care of mentally ill people requires the provision of both short and long-stay accommodation, community psychiatric care and day-care hospital. Under the Community Care Act (1990) these are a joint responsibility between the local authority and the DHA. The DHA usually ensures the responsibility for health services is met through purchasing appropriate services from health care providers. The local authority now also has a role in purchasing care in the community such as the provision of accommodation and day care for people with a chronic mental illness.

PEOPLE WITH LEARNING DISABILITIES ('MENTAL HANDICAP')

Abour four per thousand of the population have learning disabilities. Under the age of 25 years the majority live at home. In the past, those who were severely disabled or those whose families were no longer able to provide total care were looked after by health authorities in long-stay hospitals. The NHS and Community Care Act (1990) transferred to local authorities responsibility for maintaining a register of people with learning disability and for the provision of appropriate accommodation. They can do this either through local authority hostels or, more commonly, by purchasing accommodation and care from private and voluntary organizations. This has meant that the hospitals which traditionally provided care for this group stopped admissions of new long-stay patients. Consequently, the number of people in private care far outweighs those accommodated in hospital. Much of the cost for care of people with learning disabilities has been shifted from the health sector to local authorities whether they are living at home or in accommodation subsidized by the council. Most health districts have one or more special teams that liaise closely with the social services staff, educational authorities and voluntary organizations in order to plan and provide adequate services for this group.

THE COST OF THE NHS

Sources of finance

All employed people in the UK pay compulsory weekly or monthly national insurance contributions which partly finance the NHS. However, most of the cost of the NHS is met from general taxation. Other finance comes from charges to users, which include dental charges, prescription charges and charges to private patients in NHS hospitals (Fig. 20.2). The level of charges to users and the income they yield varies from time to time. Another source of funds (miscellaneous) can include the sale of NHS property, which has contributed significantly to the funding of capital programmes in the last few years though clearly this cannot continue.

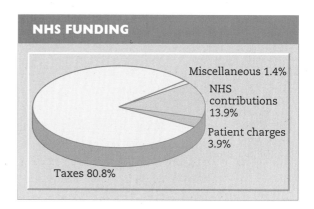

NHS FUNDING

Miscellaneous 1.4%

NHS contributions 13.9%

Patient charges 3.9%

Taxes 80.8%

Fig. 20.2 Sources of funding for the NHS, 1992/ 1993 (%).

Expenditure

In 1993/1994 the total expenditure on the NHS amounted to between 5 and 6% of the gross national product. The main categories of expenditure are shown in Fig. 20.3. Central administration costs are mainly incurred by the DoH. The expenditure of the health authorities includes the administrative costs of RHAs and DHAs. The bulk of expenditure is on purchasing all types of hospital care, community services, ambulance services, preventive medicine, health education, domiciliary nursing and health visiting and all the other provisions outlined above. Family health services expenditure includes the costs of general practitioners, pharmacists, dentists etc.

HOSPITALS

Expenditure by hospitals falls into two types:
- capital (new building and equipment);
- current (maintenance, wages and salaries, etc.).

Hospital capital expenditure

The NHS was once one of the largest property owners in the country with 1600 hospitals and nearly 50 000 acres of land. Now these assets are owned and managed by individual trusts. Trusts can buy and sell land provided they follow government procedures. The introduction of capital charging to trusts means that they have to include the true costs of capital including depreciation in their annual accounts. Proposed expenditure on new buildings has to be recorded in an annual plan and submitted to the NHS Executive for approval. Some trusts have been handicapped by inheriting old and substandard buildings. Indeed, some

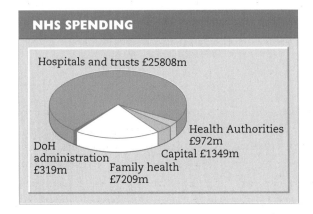

NHS SPENDING

Hospitals and trusts £25808m

Health Authorities £972m

DoH administration £319m

Capital £1349m

Family health £7209m

Fig. 20.3 NHS spending by sector 1993/1994. Total £35 657 million.

are listed buildings which puts restrictions on any alterations or modifications.

The population of some health districts has increased while others have been depopulated. As a consequence some DHAs have a surplus of hospitals beds within their area. Central London, for example, has more acute hospital accommodation than can be justified by its present resident population, although many of the hospitals there have national specialist and training functions which it is important to maintain. Closure or redeployment of beds has its own costs which will have to be met before savings can be found to use for other purposes.

Hospital current expenditure

About 65% of total hospital expenditure is on wages and salaries. This leaves little room for financial manoeuvre because the numbers of doctors, nurses and other professional staff cannot easily be adjusted to meet short-term changes in need, and cuts in this direction usually lead to a decline in services. The differences in the costs of hospitals of different types are largely due to variations in the numbers of staff that are needed to provide the services required by patients admitted, for example the clinical staff directly involved in the care of the patient, the specialist and technical staff who are necessary to enable the clinicians to function adequately (radiologists, pathologists, radiographers, scientists, laboratory technicians, operating theatre staff, intensive care staff, etc.). There are also differences between hospitals of different types in the amount of capital investment required in instruments and machinery. As manpower accounts for the major proportion of hospital costs, the weekly costs are only marginally affected by whether or not a bed is occupied or the appropriateness of its use. Thus, a chronically sick person being cared for in an acute bed costs almost the same as an acutely sick person in the same bed. Extensive misuse of hospital facilities can, if habitual, prove very wasteful.

FAMILY PRACTITIONER SERVICES
General practice

General practitioners are paid on a capitation basis (a fixed amount per year for each of the patients registered with them), supplemented by other payments including basic allowances, fees for items of service and re-imbursements for approved expenses. The FHSA has little budgetary control over the monies that it disburses although it has tried to limit pharmaceutical spending through the use of indicative prescribing amounts. Fund-holding may ultimately provide a useful way to limit general practice expenditure.

Pharmaceutical services

The FHSA expenditure on pharmaceutical services does not include the costs of drugs prescribed by hospitals, whether to in-patients or to out-patients. General practitioners write prescriptions on approved forms (FP10). These are taken by the patient or his representative to a pharmacist where they are dispensed (except in some rural areas where some general practitioners dispense their own prescriptions). There are about 11 000 pharmaceutical contractors with the NHS (one for every two general practitioners). About 300 million prescriptions are dispensed annually. The amount of money spent on the drugs prescribed by general practitioners exceeds the total expenditure on all other general medical services.

The total expenditure on different types of drugs to the NHS is affected by the basic cost of each product and the prevalence of the disease that it is designed to treat. Although the average cost of a prescription of a drug for the treatment of malignant disease is high, such drugs contribute little to the NHS drug bill because malignant disease is relatively uncommon. By contrast drugs used for the treatment of disorders of the nervous system (which are common) account for a high proportion of the drugs bill even though the average cost per prescription is low.

PLANNING HEALTH SERVICES

Objectives

The health service has no single and easily definable objective. Various facilities are provided, including specialist services for the acute sick, preventive services, primary care and care for the chronic sick and disabled. Most of the work involving direct intervention in acute sickness is purely medical in content, i.e. it is mainly dependent upon the technical skills of doctors, supported by other highly trained staff. The care of the chronic sick requires the skill mainly of other professionals, such as nurses, physiotherapists and social workers. Many preventive programmes require action by non-medical professionals, for example teachers and engineers. Health care planning is necessary in order to match needs, demands and available resources within this complex system.

RESOURCES

- Financial
- Manpower
- Facilities

Financial resources

The cost of modern medicine is now such that few people can afford to budget for it out of their income. In most countries where a state-funded system of care does not eixst, many people insure themselves against medical expenses. The difficulty about this is that the risks of long-term illnesses are difficult for a commercial company to underwrite. Even if this were possible, high premiums would have to be imposed. Chronic ill health affects the individual's earning capacity and its prevalence increases with age. Thus, the most vulnerable members of the community are the least able to maintain payment of premiums.

In order to overcome some of the obvious dangers of making each individual responsible for his or her own medical expenses, many countries have introduced health care systems that are funded either by the State or through local authorities. These either underwrite high-risk individuals or offer state-supervised and subsidized insurance. In all of these schemes, the State bears all or part of the cost from general taxation. In most, the user of services pays all or part of the cost and then reclaims a proportion from the insurance fund. This is said to be advantageous because it makes people aware of the true cost of medical care. This type of system operates in most western European countries other than the UK.

The British system is unusual in being funded from a combination of direct taxation and national insurance contributions to which are added a range of charges including prescription and dental charges. There are exemptions from charges for children, the elderly and other disadvantaged patients. Medical and other professional practitioners retain a large measure of independence, and responsible use of the service by the public is encouraged by the various charges made to patients.

Whatever the source of finance, there is a limit to the amount of money that individuals or governments can spend on health. It follows that if a high proportion of the available money is spent on one type of service, for example acute services, less is available for other important aspects of care, for example care of the chronic sick. In a state system, decisions about how the available money should be spent are political, and they must remain so, because the politicians are ultimately account-able for all public expenditure. In privately financed systems, the balance is determined by the amount of money each individual has and is willing to spend. As the working population have the greatest spending power, this usually results in a growth of acute services to the detriment of services for the elderly, the mentally ill and the disabled.

Staffing resources

The second constraint on health service planning is the numbers and types of trained personnel that are available. The principal groups involved are doctors, nurses and technicians.

Absolute manpower deficiencies arise from a shortfall in national training programmes, by net emigration of personnel, or by a need to increase the staff available to meet rapid advances in diagnostic and therapeutic technology. In the developed world, absolute deficiencies are uncommon; manpower problems result mainly from poor distribution. This occurs because:

• certain specialties may be less attractive to a young graduate than others. For example, it has always been easier to recruit general surgeons and physicians than it has been to attract people to geriatrics and psychiatry. Usually, people tend to train for specialties that interest them rather than for those that are most needed.

• some areas of the country are more desirable to live in than others; because of this there may be an overprovision in some districts and severe deficit in others.

Facilities

The availability of sophisticated equipment can restrict the development of services even if manpower and finance are adequate. This is par-ticularly important for planning the responses to new technological developments.

CHAPTER 21

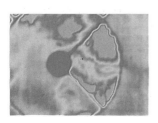

Evaluation of Health Services

INTRODUCTION

The latest health reforms in the UK were introduced in the belief that the application of the principles of the marketplace would improve both the quality and the efficiency of services. Under these reforms, purchasers have a choice of which services they wish to buy and the providers are rewarded by appropriate payment. This challenges providers to improve their quality of care in order to attract funding. If at the same time they can improve their efficiency, they are able to use the surplus funds to improve further the services they offer. It is believed that the overall standard of care will be improved by the introduction of competition. Providers need marketing skills within their organization to attract new customers and to ensure they retain current contracts. They also require detailed knowledge of both the quality of services they provide and the needs of their customers. This approach aims to ensure that provider organizations become more customer-orientated.

Purchasers require information to help them buy appropriate services on behalf of the population of their area. They need detailed demographic information concerning their population and information about local morbidity and mortality. It is intended that competition will ensure that services are provided efficiently and that costs are kept to a minimum. The purchaser must be sure that the quality of care is maintained. However, the health service is not a perfect market—certain specialist services are in short supply and when a monopoly situation arises prices may be inflated.

Whether the purchasers of services are general practitioner fundholders or DHAs, they are expected to purchase on the basis of needs. To understand needs, purchasers have to have clear aims, and have to be able to prioritize services. They may wish to concentrate on protecting the health of the population, or may wish to go further and improve health status. They may also wish to reduce current inequities in health status. Whatever their goals, purchasers are best served by purchasing effective health care. Some needs may be identified that cannot be met because effective treatments are not available or are too expensive in relation to the expected benefit. Sometimes there is a demand for care but because it is deemed that the treatments are ineffective or unnecessary they are not provided—this is sometimes thought of as a 'want' rather than a health need. Cosmetic surgery or alternative therapies are sometimes placed in this category. It must be remembered that the physical needs of patients are not the only responsibility of the health service; psychological and social needs also should be taken into account. Thus, there can be needs for support, rehabilitation or social services that help maintain and improve health.

HEALTH NEEDS

There is no absolute definition of 'need' for medical care. It is determined in part by the nature of the patient's problem, and in part by what medical services can offer. Some needs are perceived by individuals for themselves. Other needs are not perceived by individuals but may be recognized by others. Not all people who feel unwell seek professional assistance. They take action themselves, for example by going to bed for 2 days because of influenza or take advice from a friend or relative. Once they decide that they require medical intervention they make a demand on the health service. The doctor who sees the patient may or may not then accept that the problem will benefit from his or her skills. The only type of 'need' that can be measured without special study is that which creates a demand on the service.

Needs assessment

When estimating the need for health services within a population, it is useful first to look at the prevalence and incidence of the diseases concerned within the population. This coupled with the demographic data is the minimal baseline information required in order to estimate need. Interpretation of epidemiological data on need should take into account factors such as age, gender and ethnicity. It is necessary also to take into account whether an effective intervention exists, and the availability of the necessary facilities and resources to meet identified needs.

Unperceived needs

An individual who is aware of his or her need for medical intervention has symptoms or signs which he or she associates with illness. However, the professional worker may detect signs of disease that is amenable to treatment in the absence of such symptoms. This is sometimes incidental to examination for another reason or may come to light from screening or health examination surveys.

DEMANDS

The work load of a health service is affected by the incidence of acute diseases and the prevalence of chronic diseases for which care may be required over a long period. Demand is measured either by monitoring the workload of the service or by special surveys conducted in the population. Demands on services are not always an accurate proxy for need. They are affected by:

• knowledge of the existence of services;
• local availability of services;
• sectional pressure for intervention.

Without knowledge of the existence of a facility, for example total hip replacement, an individual will not make a demand for that service. He or she may, therefore, perceive a need to have the pain relieved, yet take no action. The publicity given to a particular service, for example by a television documentary, inevitably increases the perceived need and therefore increases demand. Similarly, demand is likely to be greater where a particular specialist facility is available locally and this is known to the local population and their doctors. Often demand is stimulated by local pressure groups and local media campaigns. Examples include pressure to resist closure of an accident and emergency department and campaigns to raise funds for a particular facility that has public appeal, such as a scanner for the local hospital.

QUALITY IN HEALTH CARE

Quality is a nebulous concept. It is a function of both the service provided and the expectation of the customer. Thus, as expectations rise, patients' perception of the quality of care is likely to fall. The maintenance of quality has often been focused on the elimination of bad or unacceptable practice. Increasingly, the concept of continual improvement has been adopted. This requires the structures and processes involved in health care to be continually modified, whilst careful monitoring demonstrates the improvement in outcomes. This entails the application of the so-called 'quality cycle' in which a standard of care is set, the process of care given is monitored and the outcome is measured, then new standards are adopted. Measurement of quality can involve every patient treated, as is applied, for example, to renal dialysis patients and those undergoing chemotherapy, or it can involve a sample of patients.

AUDIT

Another way of ensuring the quality of services is the use of audit. This has two aspects: medical audit and clinical audit. Medical audit refers to the assessment of care offered by doctors. Consequently, it is usually carried out by means of peer review. An audit can be undertaken when a problem or a series of problems has arisen with a particular doctor. The work and outcomes of that doctor are then examined to try to identify the reasons with a view to remedial action.

Clinical audit examines the total package of care offered to patients. This may involve assessment of the structure and process of care as well as outcomes. Clinical audit reviews not only medical care, but also nursing care, the physical environment and the organization and management of services.

EVIDENCE-BASED HEALTH CARE

Many illnesses or diseases have a range of treatments which can all be effective. Some have treatments which are unproved, or may have harmful effects in addition to their benefits. For others, there are no effective treatments. When evaluating services in an environment of limited resources, a comparison of the relative benefits and risks of available managements (including no treatment) must be made. Benefits and harm can be assessed in terms of either cost or some measure of health outcome. Much medical practice is based on anecdotal evidence and 'experience' which may be unreliable and biased. Rational decisions on which treatment options to choose are based on evidence acquired from population studies. This uses a hierarchy of evidence, with the highest quality normally ascribed to RCTs. These are not always possible, however, and in these circumstances evidence from cohort and case–control studies may be used.

A useful framework for considering the evaluation and audit of health care involves looking at the seven aspects of care outlined below.

ASPECTS OF CARE

- Efficacy: does it work?
- Effectiveness: how well does it work?
- Efficiency: is this the best way of doing it?
- Equity: is it fair?
- Accessibility: can everyone use the services?
- Acceptability: is it what they want?
- Appropriateness: is it what they need?

EFFICACY

Efficacy is the measure of the capacity of an intervention to produce a desired effect.

EFFECTIVENESS

Effectiveness involves assessing clinical outcomes of health care such as mortality rates and survival times. A treatment must show an improvement in clinical outcome, ideally through use of RCTs, in order to be considered effective.

EFFICIENCY

Efficiency involves the assessment of the costs of services. The most efficient service will produce the desired outcome at the lowest cost.

EQUITY

Equity involves assessing differences in the needs of those receiving care, differences in their treatment or differences in their outcomes to ensure that services are fairly distributed. Thus, people from minority groups or those of low socio-economic status, despite a similar or often higher prevalence of disease, may have lower rates of treatment. Even if treated on an equitable basis, outcomes may still be worse. The equity of a service can only be judged if these factors are identified and monitored. They are often only remedied by targetting of services to the disadvantaged group.

ACCESS

Access involves the assessment of barriers to care in order to ensure that people obtain the treatment they need when they need it. Barriers can include cost, waiting lists, location of the service or the need to convince a general practitioner of need. Often these barriers are only identified by asking patients directly.

ACCEPTABILITY

Acceptability Some services may not be used because of the way they are provided. Issues such as privacy, the gender or attitude of staff, and the setting of the service can influence the utilization of health services. These factors are often only discovered through patient questionnaires.

APPROPRIATENESS

Appropriateness Any assessment of health services must measure whether the needs of the population are being met. This requires constant assessment of need and audit of the structure of health services as well as monitoring such indicators as waiting lists.

ACCREDITATION

In some countries, the concept of accrediting organizations that meet certain quality standards is being adopted within the health service. Accreditation is common practice, for example in the food industry, and is sometimes applied to hospital laboratories. The assessment includes standards of practice (including the training of staff), adherence to protocols, validity and reliability of diagnostic testing, safety standards, etc. The concept of accreditation is applied to the whole range of hospital and community services in the USA and Australasia: accreditation provides purchasers with an assured quality standard which is taken into account when negotiating contracts. In many cases, accredited hospitals are rewarded by being paid a higher rate for the services they provide. UK purchasers use similar processes to monitor the quality of services provided by contractors.

HEALTH ECONOMICS

The cost of health services has been one of the Government's primary concerns since the beginning of the NHS. Management of health care costs has focused on the two principles of cost containment and efficiency. Cost containment has the disadvantage that it does not always produce improved efficiency but carries the risk of worsening outcomes.

Health economics allows an assessment of the outcomes of care to be measured against the costs by comparing one form of treatment or care with another; a decision can then be made about which is the best treatment of those compared. Several methods of comparing costs and outcomes are used.

COST EFFECTIVENESS

Cost effectiveness measures the cost of one or more treatments or services in comparison to a single outcome. Examples of outcomes that can be compared include the cost per patient successfully treated or cost per life saved. The disadvantage of a cost-effectiveness analysis is that it may not reveal other positive or negative effects of compared treatments other than those that have been recorded and which are the subject of the analysis.

COST–BENEFIT ANALYSIS

Cost–benefit analysis compares two or more treatments or services, by placing a value (usually monetary) on all the accrued costs and on all the benefits. Thus, when considering a treatment, the benefits may include added years of life. This is assigned a monetary value often based on future potential earnings of the individual. It may also include the costs of continuing care or treatment. This form of economic analysis allows purchasers to compare many different treatments to help them decide which is the best buy. The disadvantage is that it tends to discriminate against the elderly and those with a low earning potential such as the physically disabled and those with learning disabilities because the benefits are not easily measurable in monetary terms.

COST–UTILITY ANALYSIS

Cost–utility analysis accounts for all the costs of comparable treatments, but measures the benefits in a common unit (other than money). One common unit that has been used is the quality adjusted life year (QALY). A QALY combines the quantity of life gained with an adjustment for quality of life. This allows direct comparison between treatments but is less discriminatory against those with limited earning capacity than cost–benefit analysis. Other measures of the benefits of medical care have been developed, for example in 1993 the World Bank adopted a new and more sophisticated unit, disability adjusted life years (DALY).

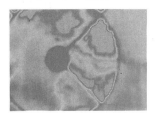

Suggested
Further Reading

Armitage P, Berry G. *Statistical Methods in Medical Research*. Oxford: Blackwell Scientific Publications, 1987.

Armstrong D. *An Outline of Sociology as Applied to Medicine*, 3rd edn. Bristol: John Wright, 1989.

Ashton J, Seymour H. *The New Public Health*. Milton Keynes: Open University Press, 1990.

Barker DJP, Rose G. *Epidemiology in Medical Practice*, 4th edn. Edinburgh: Churchill Livingstone, 1990.

Beaglehole R, Bonita R, Kjellstrom T. *Basic Epidemiology*. Geneva: World Health Organization, 1993.

Benenson AS. *Control of Communicable Disease in Man*. Washington D.C.: American Public Health Association, 1993.

Black N, Boswell D, Gray A, Murphy S, Popay J. *Health and Diseases: A Reader*. Milton Keynes: Open University Press, 1984.

Bland M. *An Introduction to Medical Statistics*. Oxford: Oxford University Press, 1987.

Cochrane AL. *Effectiveness and Efficiency: Random Reflections in Health Services*. London: British Medical Association and Nuffield Provincial Hospital Trust, 1989.

Davies RS, Fyfe C, Tannahill A. *Health Promotion: Models and Values*. Oxford: Oxford Medical Publications, 1988.

Donaldson RJ, Donaldson LJ. *Essential Public Health Medicine*. Dordrecht: Kluwer Academic Publishers, 1993.

Emond RTD, Bradley JM, Galbraith NS. *Infection*, 2nd edn. Oxford: Blackwell Scientific Publications, 1989.

Drummond MF, Maynard A. *Purchasing and Providing Cost-Effective Health Care*. Edinburgh: Churchill Livingstone, 1993.

Holland WW, Detels R, Knox G. *Oxford Textbook of Public Health*. Oxford: Oxford Medical Publications, 1991.

Jacobson B, Smith A, Whitehead M (eds). *The Nations Health: A Strategy for the 1990s*. London: King Edward's Hospital Fund for London, 1991.

Joint Committee on Vaccination and Immunisation. *Immunisation Against Infectious Diseases*. London: HMSO, 1996.

McKeown T. *The Role of Medicine*. Oxford: Basil Blackwell, 1980.

Miller DL, Farmer RDT. *Epidemiology of Diseases*. Oxford: Blackwell Scientific Publications, 1982.

Richards IDG, Baker MR. *Epidemiology and Prevention of Important Diseases*. London: Churchill Livingstone, 1988.

Rose G. *The Strategy of Preventive Medicine*. Oxford: Oxford Medical Publications, 1992.

Sackett DL, Haynes RB, Guyatt GH, Tugwell P. *Clinical Epidemiology—A Basic Science for Clinical Medicine*. Boston: Little, Brown and Company, 1991.

Townsend P, Davidson N. *Inequalities in Health (The Black Report)*. London: Penguin Books, 1992.

Waldron HA. *Lecture Notes on Occupational Medicine*, 4th edn. Oxford: Blackwell Scientific Publications, 1990.

Whitehead M. *Inequalities in Health (The Health Divide)*. London: Pelican Books, 1992.

Index